Sourdough Modern Recipes for Beginners 2021

Guide for Beginners to Make Artisan Bread at Home

© Copyright 2021 - All rights reserved.

This content is provided with the sole purpose of providing relevant information on a specific topic for which every reasonable effort has been made to ensure that it is both accurate and reasonable. Nevertheless, by purchasing this content you consent to the fact that the author, as well as the publisher, are in no way experts on the topics contained herein, regardless of any claims as such that may be made within. As such, any suggestions or recommendations that are made within are done so purely for entertainment value. It is recommended that you always consult a professional prior to undertaking any of the advice or techniques discussed within.

This is a legally binding declaration that is considered both valid and fair by both the Committee of Publishers Association and the American Bar Association and should be considered as legally binding within the United States.

The reproduction, transmission, and duplication of any of the content found herein, including any specific or extended information will be done as an illegal act regardless of the end form the information ultimately takes. This includes copied versions of the work both physical, digital and audio unless express consent of the Publisher is provided beforehand. Any additional rights reserved.

Furthermore, the information that can be found within the pages described forthwith shall be considered both accurate and truthful when it comes to the recounting of facts. As such, any use, correct or incorrect, of the provided information will render the Publisher free of responsibility as to the actions taken outside of their direct purview. Regardless, there are zero scenarios where the original author or the Publisher can be deemed liable in any fashion for any damages or hardships that may result from any of the information discussed herein.

Additionally, the information in the following pages is intended only for informational purposes and should thus be thought of as universal. As befitting its nature, it is presented without assurance regarding its prolonged validity or interim quality. Trademarks that are mentioned are done without written consent and can in no way be considered an endorsement from the trademark holder

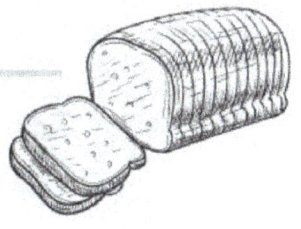

Contents

[Chapter 1: Introduction](#)
[Sourdough Starter](#)
[Tips to Keep Your Sourdough Starter](#)
[Healthy Modern Craving Sourdough](#)
[Special Oat Sourdough](#)
[Malt Sourdough](#)
[Potato Sourdough](#)
[Honey Wheat Sourdough](#)
[Rosemary with Olive Sourdough](#)
[American Style Sourdough](#)
[Cheese and Sesame Sourdough](#)
[Wheat Malted Sourdough](#)
[White Sourdough Bread](#)
[Asian Sourdough Bread](#)
[Yeast Sourdough](#)
[Eastern Wheat Sourdough](#)
[Carrot Milky Sourdough](#)
[Dark Beer Rye Sourdough](#)
[Mexican Sourdough](#)
[Cheddar Sourdough](#)
[Danish Sourdough](#)
[Milky Grain Sourdough](#)
[Spicy Jalapeno Sourdough](#)
[White, Whole Wheat Sourdough](#)
[Garlic Onion Sourdough](#)

Modern Salty Sourdough
Buckwheat Delicious Sourdough
Westerham Farm Sourdough
Ciabatta Sourdough
Hearth Flaxseed Sourdough
Light Onion Rye Sourdough
Wholegrain Sourdough
Ripped Pumpkin Sourdough
Rich Egg and Butter Sourdough
Spelt Walter Sourdough
Extra Sour Sourdough
Berlin Style Sharp
Sour Malt Sourdough
Kalamata Asiago Sourdough
Cracked Wheat Borough Sourdough
Northwestern Sourdough
Rosemary Potato Sourdough
Sourdough Hercules
Sunrise Sourdough
Honey Butter Sourdough
Lentil with Wheat Flour Sourdough
Wheaten Houston Sourdough
Hoochie Mama Sourdough
Molasses Wheat Sourdough
Francisco Sourdough
Gluten-Free Nuts sourdough
Yeast wood Sourdough
Sourdine Sourdough

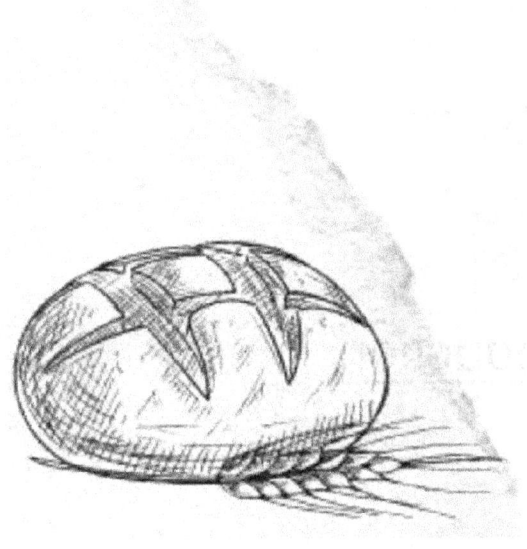

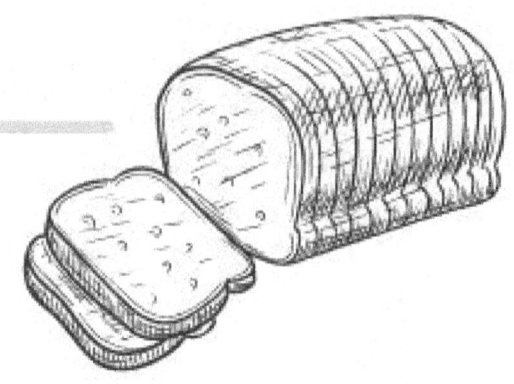

Chapter 1: Introduction

Sourdough can raise bread normally, meaning it's made without adding yeast. Wild yeast will develop by making a starter that will raise bread normally. As opposed to its name, Sourdough bread isn't always acrid tasting. Pundit more often than not will create a tart or unpleasant style chiefly because of the parts of a sourdough starter anyway. The tart taste can be changed when it arrives at the most preparing method. The underlying advance to be a sourdough pastry specialist, you should initially deliver a starter. A starter is a hitter that you'll keep in your refrigerator for quite a while. The starter that you may cause will be blended into a batter, making the bread rise. Most people believe that their sourdough starter is alive. In reality, that can be considered since a starter might be a player loaded up with yeast and microbes. It contains a lactobacillus culture in the harmonious Combine with the yeast. It's a raising for bread. Since it is a cultured yeast, it is a characteristic raising strategy. It isn't unprecedented for a pastry specialist's starter Mixture to possess long stretches of history from numerous huge loads of past clumps. Thus, every pastry kitchen's sourdough incorporates a particular taste. The blend of starter measures, reward proportions and rest times, culture and air temperature, mugginess, and height makes each cluster of sourdough extraordinary. At present, to frame the sourdough bread, you need to Combine the starter with flour to make the batter. You can make various kinds of bread, flapjacks, and cakes utilizing sourdough.

The pleasant issue concerning sourdough is that you'll store it inside the fridge however long you need (it develops besides) and make a batter at whatever point you need to. It's not tedious and simple to orchestrate. Sourdough is a sort of bread, which is made without utilizing business yeast. Rather it is made from a starter culture prepared from blending water and flour and left to age throughout some period. The maturation sum some of

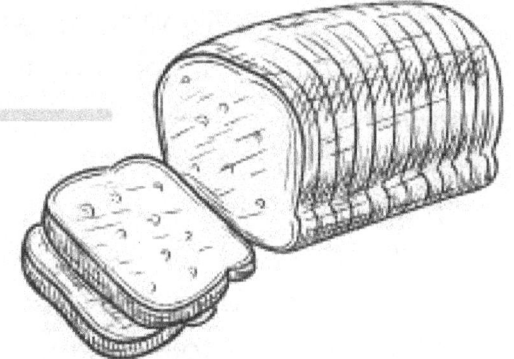

the time keeps going regarding consistently and all through this period, the way of life should be recharge consistently with more flour and warmth water. It's also called 'taking care of'. The starter is best continued during a glass container or compartment with a got top. It's prepared when it has practically twofold in volume, 'effervescent' looking with an unmistakable acidic fragrance exuding from the combination. There are a few sourdoughs plans out there; however, sourdough joins a secretive bound side concerning it. There are a few factors that affect sourdough bread-making measures Such some flour, where it comes from, the sort of water utilized, the season, and even area all joins an addressing the starter culture and the genuine portion. A formula is exclusively a guide. A sourdough portion that has been prepared and tried in a mechanical kitchen will regularly have an entirely unexpected look and character when heated in an extremely homegrown kitchen.

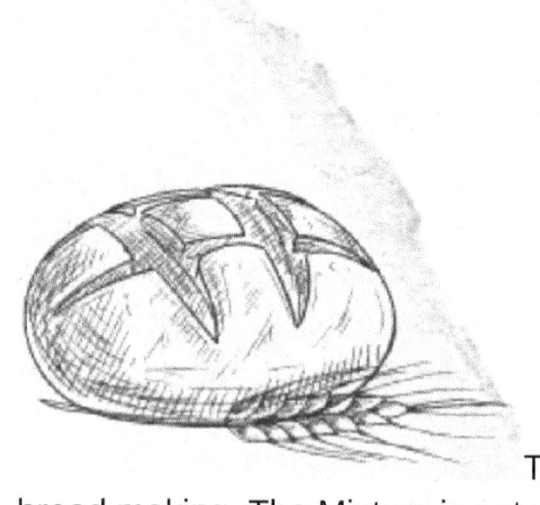

There is likewise no easy route to sourdough bread making. The Mixture is set up by blending a portion of the starter culture with heat water, flour of option (rye, spelled, wholemeal unbleached, solid premium white, or a Combine of many), and ocean salt. Entirely unexpected flour will turn out portion with great character, surface, and taste. This is trailed by a progression of massaging and resting over a measure of numerous hours - between six to eight hours depending on the season or potentially surrounding temperature of the space. Broiler temperatures also assume a significant part in the result. A low warmth will fabricate sourdough bread with a thicker hull. Everything broilers don't appear to be made indistinguishable. Acquaintance with the stove and its personality would be an extraordinary benefit with regards to sourdough preparation. Regularly it may take extra than one endeavor to supply the ideal portion. The proverb "apply makes great" is the way into the craft of sourdough bread making. Sourdough conjointly makes the radiant base for pizza, pies, and elective sweet or flavorful treats requiring bake good sod like tarts. While making most kinds of bread, you need fixings like flour, water, salt, and a raising specialist. You blend everything along, let it rest for though structure it, leave

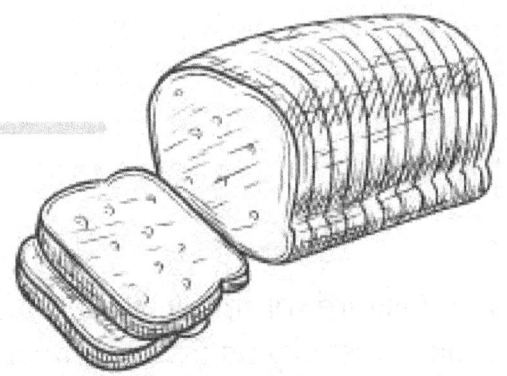

it for a while, and it readied to prepare. Sourdough is entirely unexpected. While it requires every one of the most fixings like all unique bread, it is made without using a raising specialist. It is one among the most seasoned sorts of bread, tracing back to Ancient Egypt. Since sourdough bread is made without the enhancement of cook's yeast, the yeast must be filled in an incredibly sourdough starter. This wild yeast developed inside the starter is the thing that gives sourdough bread its novel taste. Making sourdough bread isn't burdensome either; first of all, a starter requires to be made, the fixings are water and flour. You join heat water and flour and leave it in a dull spot. At that point, each day, discard 0.5 of the starters and add new water and flour. After a while, your starter will have developed a significant touch. As you can see by right now, making sourdough bread exclusively needs persistence. Mind your starter time from time, and it

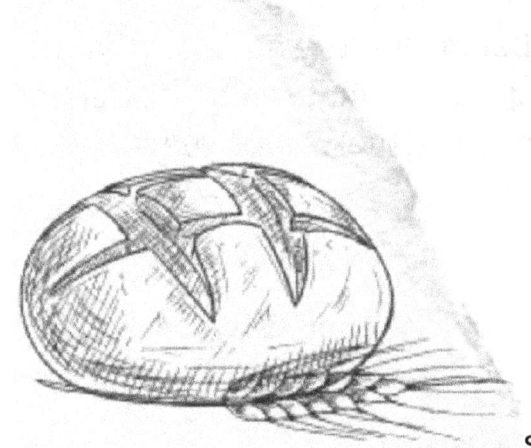

should have a severe smell that looks like brew. Before you might want to heat your sourdough, bread place the starter during a container, essentially make positive that it isn't impermeable, the wild yeast inside the starter could be a living creature and needs air to live. Store it in a cool and dull spot; don't store it in heat places as the warmth will murder the yeast. Try not to utilize metallic compartments as they will influence the flavor of your bread quickly.

Sourdough Starter

A sourdough starter is a Mixture or hitter that contains wild yeasts and microbes, has an observable causticity as an aftereffect of maturation by these creatures, and is utilized to raise different batters. A sourdough starter is additionally called a characteristic sharp or regular starter. Before industrially arranged yeast was out there, bread was begun by blending flour and water and allowing this combination to remain till wild yeasts started to age it. This starter was then used to raise bread. A segment of the starter was saved, blended in with more flour and water, and put aside to present the following day's bread. This strategy stays utilized nowadays. Sourdough is a very bread made without the utilization of cook's yeast, and it raises by

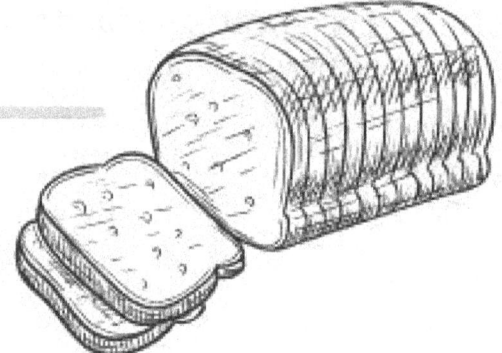

developing common yeast, which gives it its unmistakable severe style. Sourdough has been made for millennia before there was grown yeast, likely beginning in Ancient Egypt. A sourdough starter that can be utilized for making the Mixture as of now wants to be made to develop wild yeast.

You will require water, found a compartment for the capacity of your sourdough starter. First, pick a room with a seal. An item like Tupperware is reasonable; however, a glass container with a seal will be utilized comparably well. Avoid using metal compartments as they will change the style of the sourdough. When you have a holder for your starter, get some warm water and some flour and empty them along into the compartment. The sourdough starter ought to be kept at room temperature. Underneath these conditions,

the yeast will develop best, use alert not to open it to temperatures over ninety (thirty-two), that could slaughter the yeast and thwart the bread from rising by and by. Consistently take 0.5 of the sourdough starters, discard them, and add a large portion of some water and some flour. Continue to do this for the resulting not many days, when a couple of days there ought to be bubbles framing, in a harsh smell. At the point when the outside of your sourdough starter gets covered with bubbles, your starter is finished. To store your sourdough starter, place a cover on your compartment that won't close it and store it during a dull and cold spot, in a perfect world, a fridge. When the starter is cooled, adding water and flour shouldn't be done extra than once each week. On the off chance that you hold your sourdough starter in the refrigerator, there is a high probability that a dull fluid can develop. This fluid contains liquor and has a singer-like smell. If your sourdough starter appearance dry, you should blend it back in, yet on the off chance that it looks wet enough, you'll have the option to spill it out. After you caused the starter,

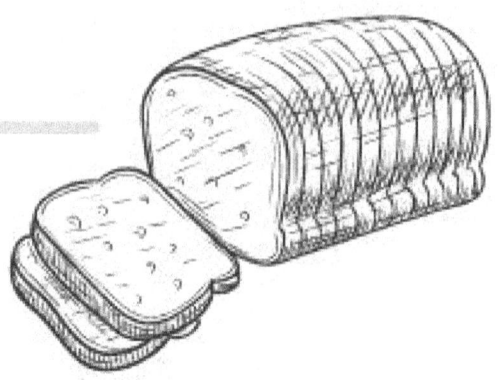

you'll to likewise need to make a bowl of hitter. When you might want to make it, you should remove the starter from the more relaxed a couple of hours sooner and spot it in a too bowl. When the compartment you utilize for the sourdough starter is unfilled, you'll subsequently wash and dry it. It's ready for use sometime later. Presently add some water and some flour to the bowl and blend everything along. When you are done, you placed the bowl with the mixture in a hot spot and licensed it to mature for a long time. When the outside of the Combine gets covered with air pockets, and there's a harsh smell, it's finished. The flavor of the bread will depend on the length

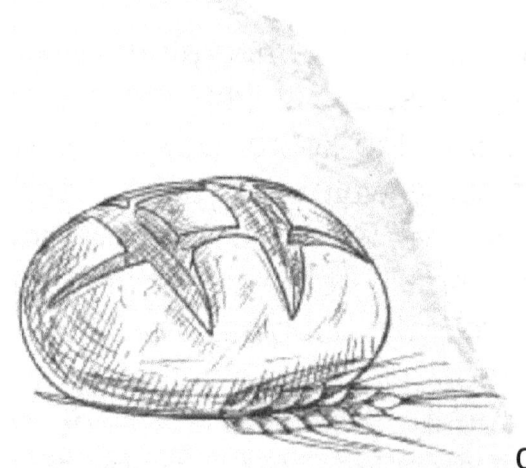

of aging. The more you let it mature, the sourer the taste can be.

Tips to Keep Your Sourdough Starter Healthy

Keeping a sourdough starter might be similar to focus on a pet or a youngster. They need legitimate conditions to flourish, you need to take care of them every day (or week by week whenever refrigerated), and they bite the dust on you if you disregard them.

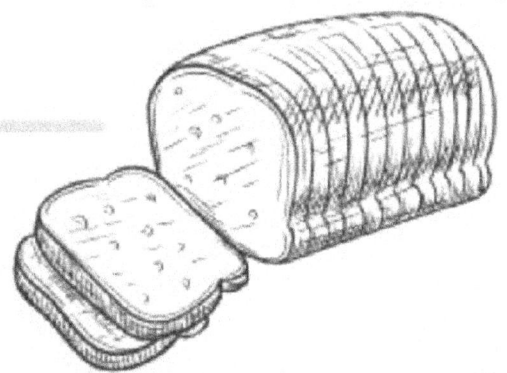

Sourdough starters need to be taken care of in any event, double each day whenever put away at room temperature, and every 3-four days whenever put away in the fridge. The more established sourdough books that teach you to add fixings to your starter, similar to the extra Mixture, late bread rolls, milk, nectar, and so on, are unfashionable. If you add anything other than water and flour to your starter, you're requesting trouble. Who knows about what microbes, yeasts, or various microorganisms from such increments can do to the great starter you as of now have? On the off chance that you feed your starter with flour and water each time, it will be predictable in its yield and maturing times. You won't acquaint an obscure segment with the starter that could, without a doubt, murder or defile it with something that can back it off or make it debilitated. Different avenues regarding adding different things to your starter, just eliminate some starter and put it into another holder to try different things with. I even have perused of experimenters adding sugar, organic product or taking care, of their starters with entirely unexpected kinds of flours or fixings. Experimentation can be fun, essentially cause positive to will free of the starter you're trying different things with from the first starter and let your unique starter be. I, for one favor starters, took care of with exclusively flours and water (juice can be utilized the initial not many days to encourage a starter going).

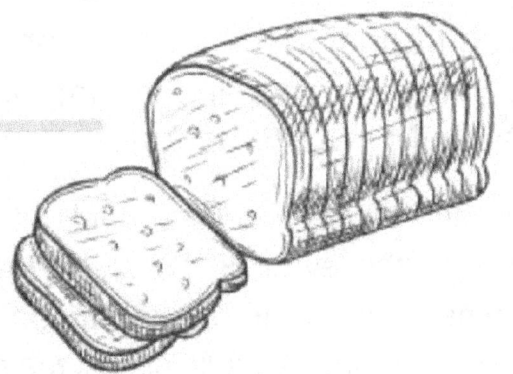

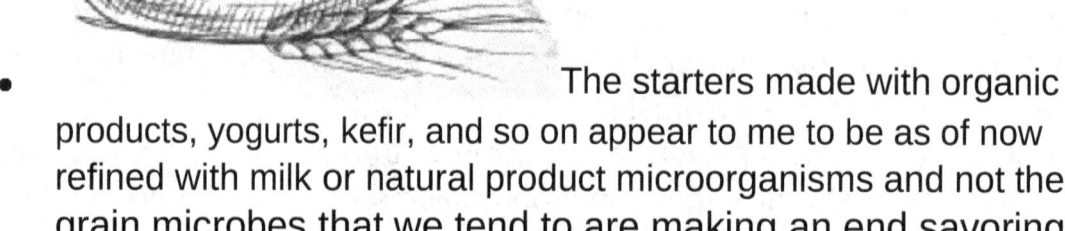

- The starters made with organic products, yogurts, kefir, and so on appear to me to be as of now refined with milk or natural product microorganisms and not the grain microbes that we tend to are making an end savoring
- I wish to draw out the style of wheat, rye, and entire grains. Not taking care of the sourdough starter often or utilizing the starter when it isn't satisfactorily revived/took care of could be a typical disadvantage, particularly for

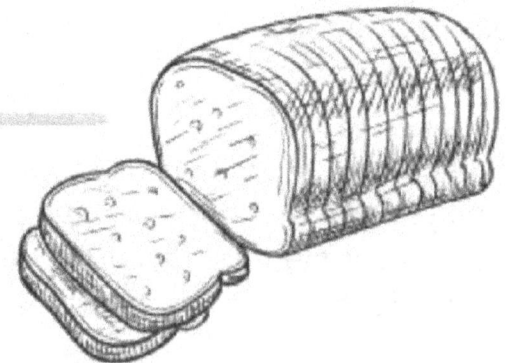

those new to sourdough heating. Additionally, you would join a huge proportion of a blend in that the gluten was de-raised, urging the Mixture to be frail.

- Feed your sourdough start regularly if hat it is at territory temperature. In the event If it inside the fridge, invigorate it a couple of times before util before stirring up the Mixture. If the starter smells horrendously acidic, spill the majority of it out and construct it back up by taking care of it a greater proportion of flour/water before util before framing the Mixture. A 166p starter.c hydration and taken care of with a lower proportion of feed to starter cannot ceaselessly look effervescent when it is set up to utilize.

- For the most part, it can look dead. By a lower proportion of feed to the starter, I imply that the amount of the starter player is bigger than the measure of feed it gets. For example, if you have two mugs of ready starter, and you feed it with one mug of water/flour combination, it won't show as a plentiful movement as though you had one mug of ready starter and you feed it with two mugs of water/flour blend.

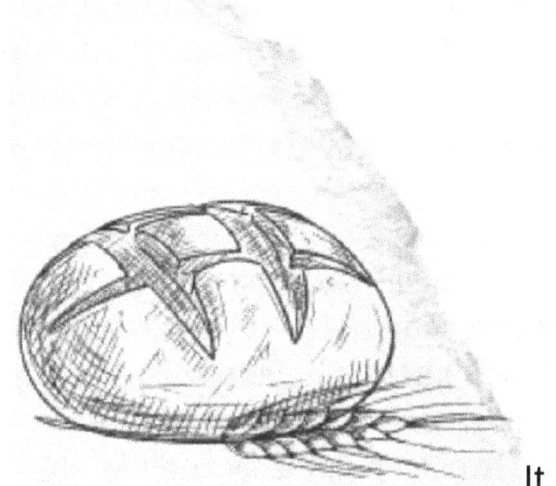

- It can astound you at how vivacious it genuinely is, in any event, when its appearance dormant. A fluid starter took care of with a goliath amount of feed may show a decent layer of thin air pockets the morning when taking care of, though the starter with a lower measure of feed couldn't show any movement.

At the point when you feed it excessively low of an amount for a really le of your time, it will, in the end, not be as dynamic or solid. Starters can be tormented by helpless water quality. The pastry shop across the cove from me had issues for quite a long time with not having the option to utilize the wild yeasts in light of helpless water quality. I sent them some of my Northwest starter she principal clump passed on. I posed them a few inquiries about the starter care and uncovered they were utilizing city fixture water to take care of the starter and fabricate the batter. Town water has chlorine and various synthetics in it, which

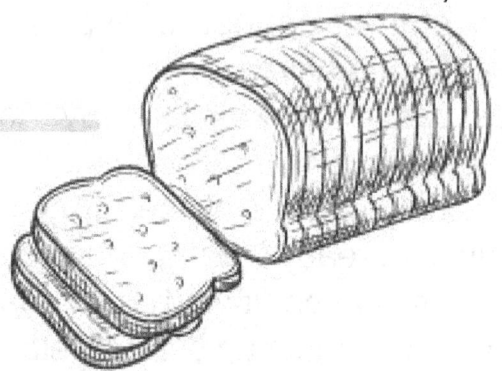

will be deadly to sourdough yeasts. The pastry kitchen has been effectively heating incredible sourdough since separating their water. Other than chlorine, there may be different synthetic substances in city spigot water that can hurt sourdough yeasts. Locate the best water you'll and use it for both taking care of the starter and for making up the Mixture. Separated water is commonly acceptable. Water that has been refined isn't the least difficult for sourdough preparing because the salts and minerals have been taken out and that they not exclusively help to take care of the yeasts and microorganisms, anyway, conjointly influence the kind of water (and the bread). Nonetheless, refined water keeps on being desirable over unfiltered faucet water. On the off chance that faucet water is all that is effectively available to you, heat the water, cool it, and afterward empty it into a compartment that you'll have the option to keep approximately covered. This way, some of the unstable gasses have a likelihood to disseminate. Leave the holder inexactly lined for 24 - 48 hours. At that point, cover and store it to be utilized in taking care of your starter and the blending of your Mixture. The utilization of bubbled fixture water has been fruitful for those that exclusively have faucet water reachable to them or on the off chance that they don't have a clue what may be inside the water, as in little or non-public well water sources. I have heard that a few people have had no issues utilizing their fixture water with sourdough pre-preparation to remunerate a starter that looks or scents dubious eliminates concerning one-fourth mug of the starter, and it put aside in a spotless bowl. Dispose of the remainder of the starter and clean the starter compartment truly well, scratching down the edges and clothing with high temp water. Try not to utilize blanch or cleanser, basically high temp water. At that point, add back the one-fourth mug of held starter and begin taking care of it again. Whenever you have the starter working out in a good way, keep it in the cooler

(an enthusiastic

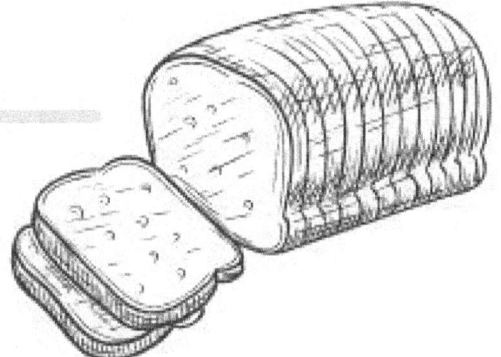

little residence fridge kept between 42 - 48 degrees are ideal) on the off chance that the temperature too heat, you will not take care of it as a rule, especially on the off chance that you don't prepare all the time.

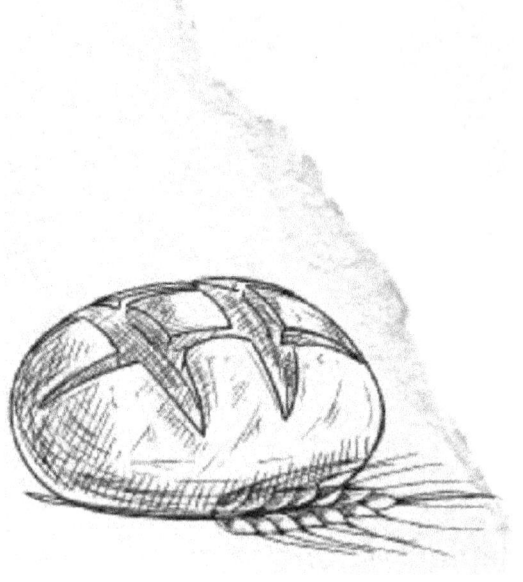

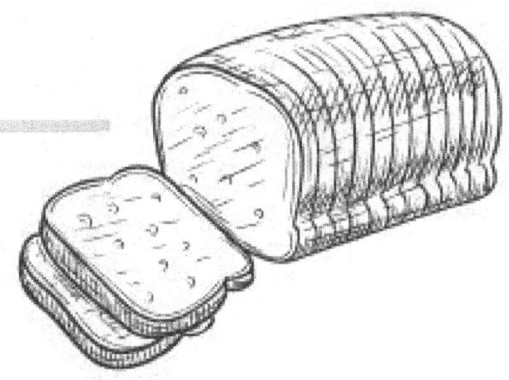

Modern Craving Sourdough

Ingredients:

- 1 mug (240 ml) water
- 1 teaspoon salt
- Makes one 1half-pound (680 g) loaf
- Mug (240 ml) culture from the Culture Proof
- 3half mugs (490 g) unbleached all-purpose flour

Instructions:

- Place the shaped loaf during a bread pan or different baking container, in a willow basket, or, for French loaves, on a baking sheet. Cover and proof (either at room temperature or in the warmer atmosphere of a proofing box, depending on your preferred temperature) for two to 4 hours until it has doubled in bulk or reached nearly to the high of the bread pan. Remember that proofing at higher temperatures (ninety/thirty twoc) can produce a sourer loaf with smart flavor but decreased
- leavening. Proofing at area temperature can yield smart leavening and delicate sourness. Proofing at room temperature for the primary hour, and then at ninety (thirty-two) can yield a moderately bitter loaf with only slightly decreased leavening. Just before putting the loaf within the oven, slash the surface of the dough many times with a razor blade. Place the pan with its formed, proofed loaf in an exceedingly cool oven, then turn the temperature to 375degrees Fahrenheit (one hundred ninety) and bake for 70 minutes.
- Or transfer the loaf to a preheated baking stone in a very

450degrees Fahrenheit(230°C) oven and bake for forty minutes. For a firm, chewy crust, place a pan of boiling water below the loaf or spritz the oven

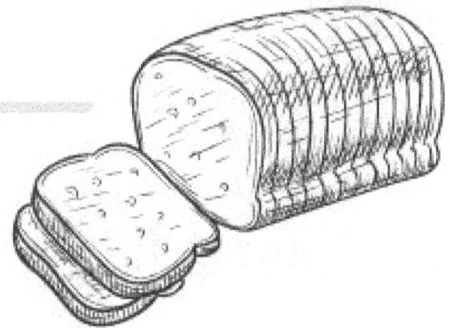

with water every five minutes for fifteen minutes whereas the oven is at baking temperature. When the loaf is baked, remove it from the pan and let cool on a wire rack for a minimum of 15 to 20 minutes before slicing.

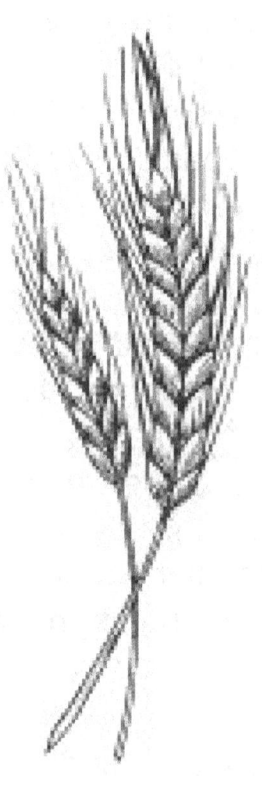

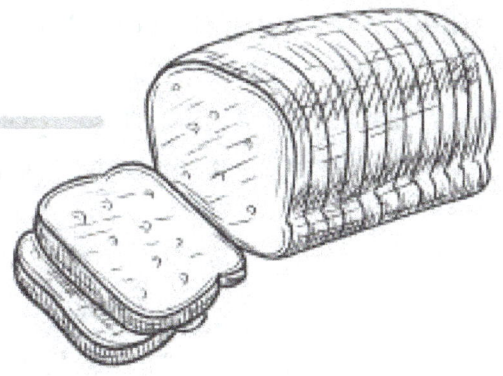

Special Oat Sourdough

Ingredients

- room temperature 2 apples, peeled and
- grated 1 mug (200 ml) rolled oats one-
- fourth mug (50 ml) water,

Instructions:

- Combine the oats during a blender until they reach a consistency simply like flour. Combine the ingredients and let them rest two-four days with a smart-fitting lid. Stir inside the mornings and evenings. The starter is prepared when the Mixture starts to bubble. From now on, all you've got to try and do is "feed" the dough therefore that it retains its flavor and ability to ferment.

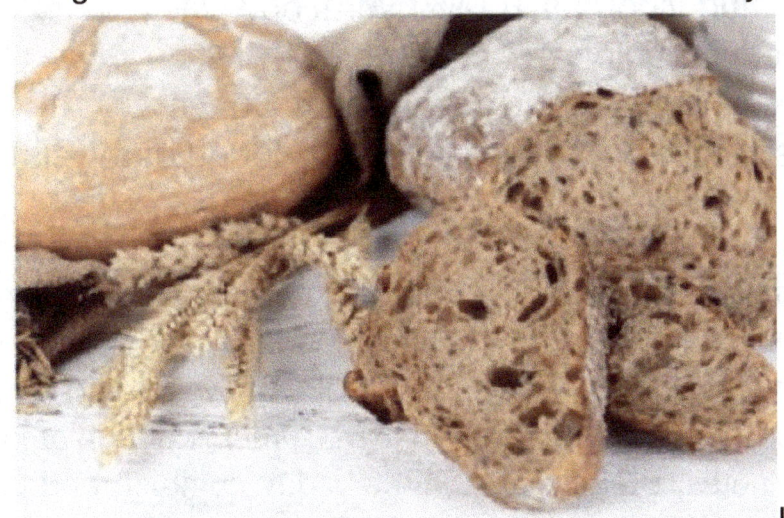

- If you allow the sourdough within the refrigerator, you ought to feed it once per week with a half mug (100 ml) water and one mug (100 g) oat flour. If you retain the sourdough at space temperature, it should be fed every day, identically. The consistency ought to resemble thick porridge. If you have got sourdough left over, you may be ready to freeze it in containers that hold a mug.

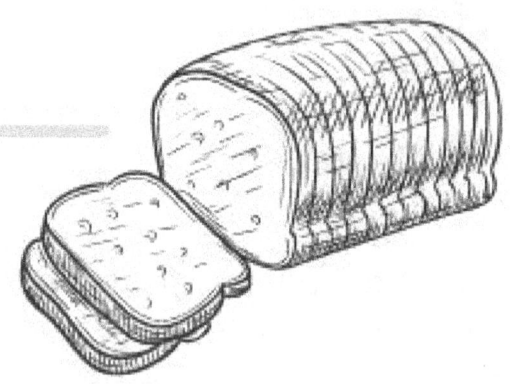

Malt Sourdough

Ingredients:

- 2 mugs water– 16.0 Ounce
- half mug evaporated canned milk – 4.0 Ounce
- 2 Tbsp malt syrup or honey - 1.6 Ounce 2
- Tbsp melted, cooled butter- 1Ounce
- 3/4 mug vigorous 100% hydration Rye
- sourdough starter – 6.7 Ounce
- 8 mugs Bread flour – 2-pound 4 Ounce
- 4 tsp salt – .8 Ounce (add after dough autolysis)

Instructions:

- Combine all of the ingredients (except the salt) well in your Mixer for concerning two – 3 minutes on low speed or just until combined. Then enable the dough autolysis (rest) for 20 minutes.
- After autolysis, add salt and then Combine dough at low speed for 5 minutes. Bread made with a 1 day combine and bake formula need to be combined longer to develop the gluten. Allow the dough to bulk ferment (that just suggests that the first rise) for four hours. Stir the dough down with just 3 turns of the

dough hook twice throughout the 4-hour bulk fermentation. This is to strengthen the gluten strands and line them up, much like folding would do. You'll additionally put the dough into a dough folding trough and fold the dough twice throughout bulk ferment. Dough made with rye flours tends to be sticky.

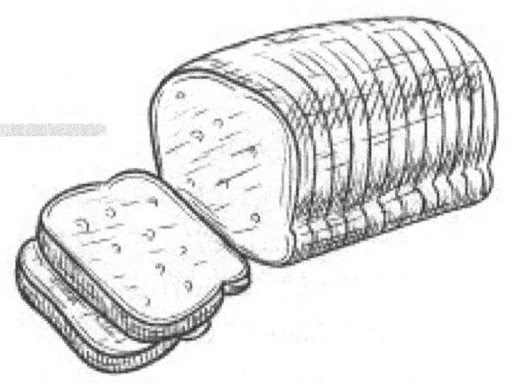

Potato Sourdough

Ingredients:

- Two medium size
- peeled 1 tsp honey 1 tbsp spelled flour, sifted

Instructions:

- Combine the potatoes till they resemble gruel. Stir inside the honey and spelled flour. Store the Mixture in an exceeding jar with a decent-fitting lid. Stir in the mornings and evenings. This sourdough typically takes a very little longer to make than others, however, it's valuing

the extra time. It will take 5-seven days before it's done. The starter is ready when the mixture bubble.

- From now on, all you have got Sourdine to do is "feed" the dough so that it retains its flavor and talent to ferment. If you leave the sourdough within the refrigerator, you must feed it once per week with a half mug (100mammall potato gruels and one to spelled you keep the sourdough anathema rea temperature, it ought to be fed each day, in the identical consistency must resemble thick porridge. If you've got sourdough left over, you'll be in a position to freeze it in containers that hold 0. five a mug.

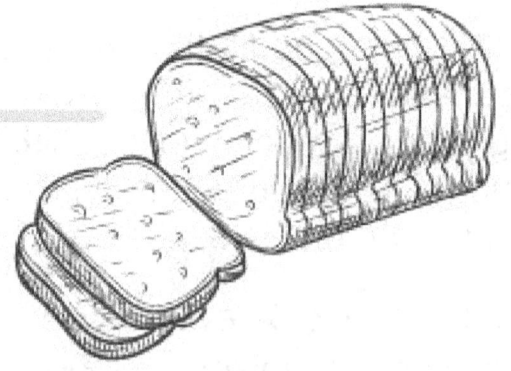

Honey Wheat Sourdough
Ingredients:

- 9 mugs (1.1 kg) wheat flour
- mugs (500 ml) water, room temperature

- 12 Ounce (350 g) wheat sourdough starter
- two-third mug (150 g) water, room
- temperature mugs (250 g) wheat flour
- 1third-fourth tsp (5 are fourth tsp half –1 tbsp
- honey half tbsp (10 g) salt

Instructions:

- To the dough that was prepared the day before, add all ingredients except the salt. Knead until the dough is elastic, then add the salt. Shape the dough into three round loaves by dividing it into thirds.

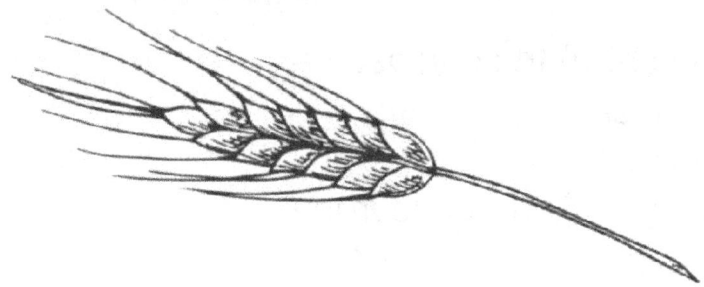

- Place the loaves on a greased baking sheet after gently dipping them in flour. Allow the loaves to rise for about 10 hours in the refrigerator. Preheat the oven to 475degrees Fahrenheit(240°C) and bake the loaves for 25–30 minutes.

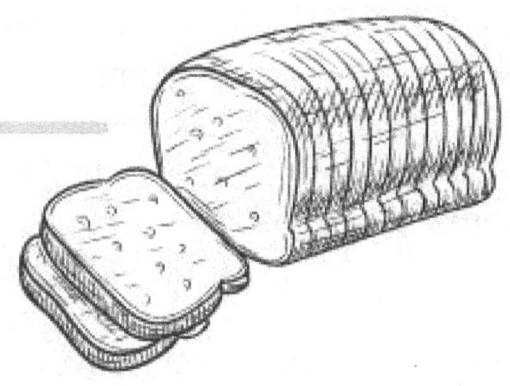

Rosemary with Olive Sourdough

Ingredients:

- 3half tsp (10 g) fresh yeast
- 1 tsp (5 g) salt
- 1 tbsp olive oil
- 1 Ounce (80 g) wheat sourdough starter
- 2 mugs (250 g) wheat flour
- half mug (125 ml) water, room
- temperature fresh rosemary

Instructions:

- Combine all the ingredients, except the oil and rosemary, until you've got a swish dough. Let it rise for twenty minutes. Roll out the dough and shape it into a rectangle that's regarding one-tenth of an in. (three mm) thick. Brush with olive oil. Chop the rosemary and sprinkle on high of the dough. Then, roll the dough up from the short facet of the rectangle. Secure the ends. Let the bread rise for regarding thirty minutes and score a deep incision in the middle of the dough roll thus that each one of the layers is visible.
- Let it rise for an additional 10 minutes. Initial oven temperature: 475degrees Fahrenheit(250°C) Place the bread among the oven rankle a mug of water onto the bottom of the oven. Lower the temperature to four hundred (210°C) and bake for concerning 20 minutes. Brush the dough with oil and unfold the rosemary evenly on

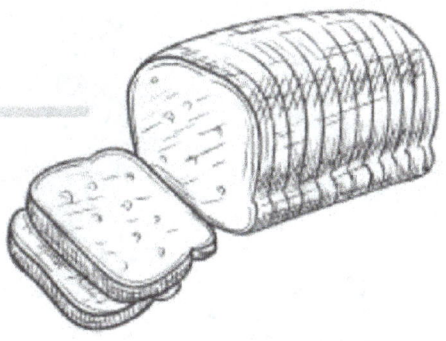

prime. Roll the dough up. Pinch the ends of along. Score the bread when it's risen.

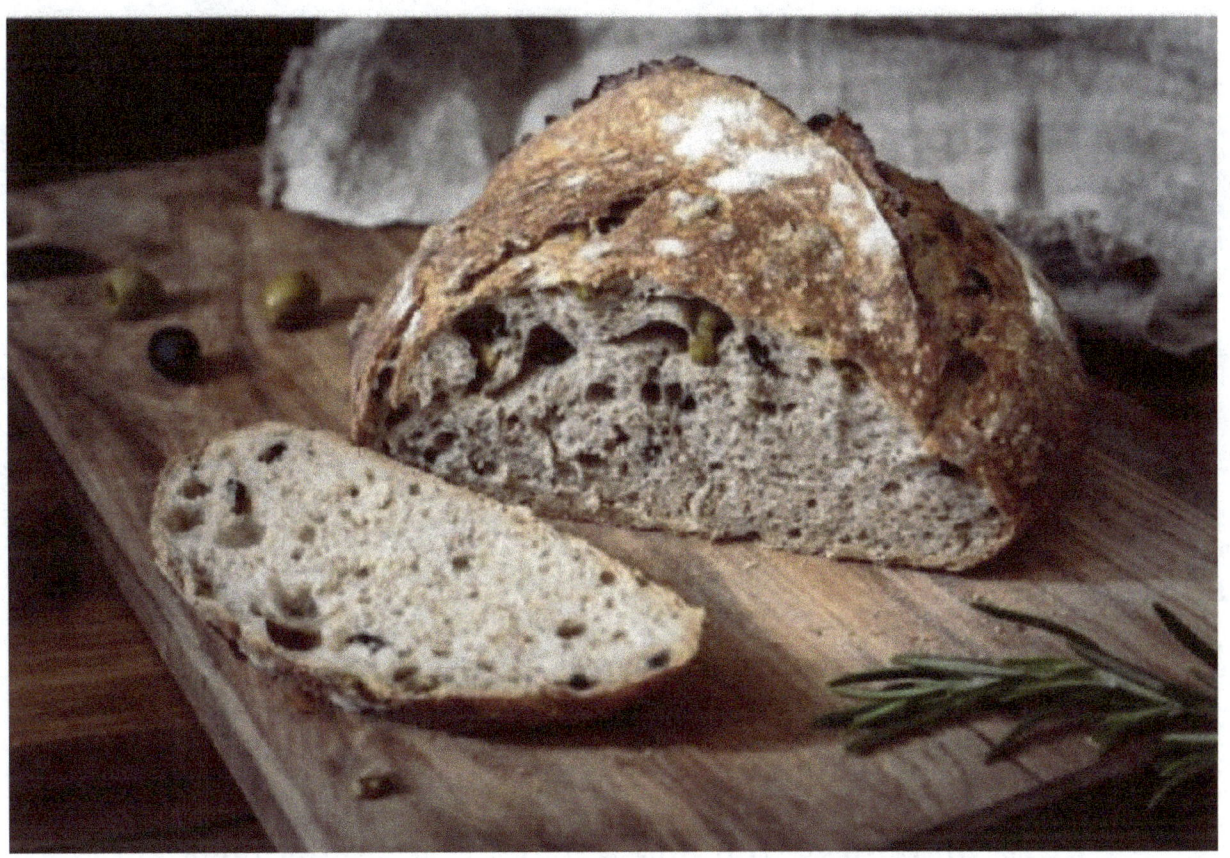

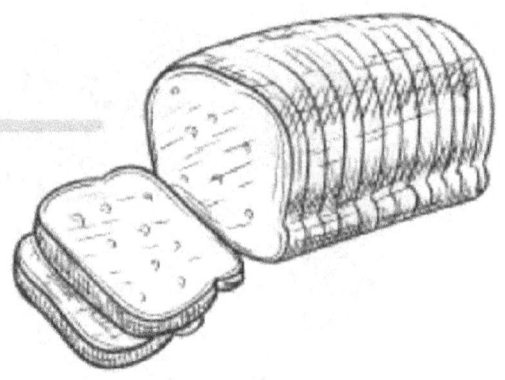

American Style Sourdough

Ingredients:

- 1half tsp salt
- 1 mug (240 ml) water
- Makes one 1half-pound (680 g) loaf
- 1 mug (240 ml) culture from the culture proof
- 3half mugs (490 g) unbleached all-purpose flour

Instructions:

- Empty the way of life into a blending bowl. Break down the salt in the water and Combine it into the way of life. Add the flour to a mug at an at once tilt's too solid to even consider consolidating with a spoon. Turn out onto a floured board and massage inside the leftover flour till the batter is smooth and silken. Or on the other hand blend and ply the entirety of the elements for the greater part of 25 minutes in a bread machine or other.
- After the thirty-minute rest, shape the batter. Smooth it marginally, at that point raise some from the outskirts and pull it toward the middle. Proceed with this round the Mixture mass to frame a harsh ball, at that point structure as a French portion by tenderly tapping the batter into an unpleasant square shape, at that point collapsing over and squeezing the edges along to shape a crease.
- Spot the formed portion, crease side down, on a preparing sheet confirmation, for two to four hours till it duplicates in mass. For a reasonable Combine of acridity and raising, evidence the portion for the essential hour at space temperature and afterward

at eighty-five° to ninety (29° to thirty twoc) in a very sealing box. Spot the preparing sheet with its shaped portion in a cool stove, at that point flip the

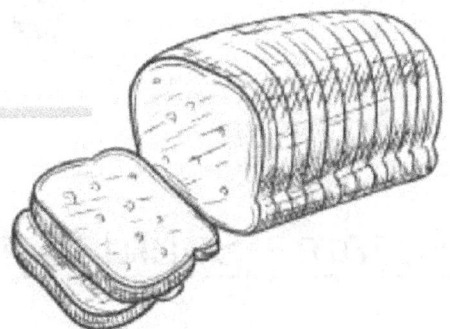

temperature to 375degrees Fahrenheit (a hundred ninety) and heat for 70 minutes. Or then again move the portion to a preheated preparing stone in a 450degrees Fahrenheit(230°C) stove and heat for forty minutes.

- For a firm, chewy outside layer, place a container of bubbling water underneath the portion or spritz the broiler with water every 5 minutes for 15 minutes while the stove is at heating temperature. At the point when the portion is prepared, eliminate it from the container and let it cool on a wire rack for at least fifteen to 20 minutes prior before.

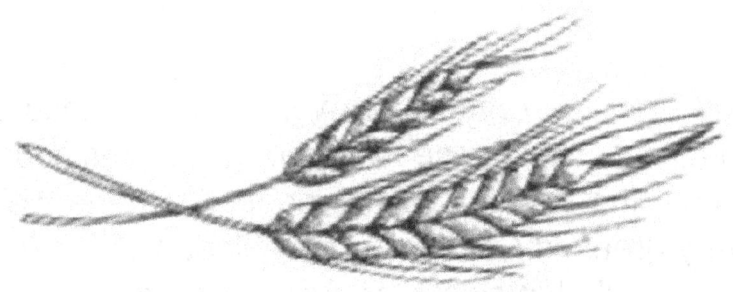

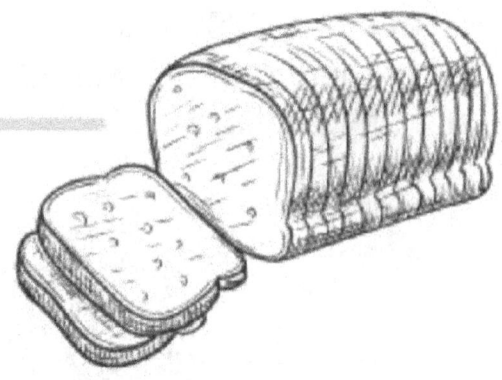

Cheese and Sesame Sourdough

Ingredients:

- 1half mug (350 ml) water, room temperature
- 1half mug (200 g) durum wheat flour
- 1half mug (200 g) wheat flour
- 1 tbsp (15 g) salt
- 2one-fourth mug (250 g) grated cheese, such as aged Swiss or Emmental
- half mug (100 ml) toasted sesame seeds
- 8half Ounce (240 g) wheat sourdough starter
- 3two-third mugs (400 g) wheat flour (amount will vary depending on the cheese used)
- olive oil for the bowl

Instructions:

- Remove the dough from the refrigerator well before to ensure that it's not too cold. Add salt, cheese, sesame seeds, and flour. The drier the cheese, the less flour you'll need. Combine well and let rise in a very greased Combining bowl lined with tin foil until the dough has doubled in size. Carefully unfold the dough out on a table and cut it into thirds.
- Gently shape into spherical loaves. Place the loaves on a greased baking sheet and let the bread rise for concerning 30 minutes. Initial Oven Temperature: 450 Degrees Fahrenheit (230°C) Put the bread within the oven and cut back the temperature to 400

degrees Fahrenheit (210°C). Bake for regarding notes Toasts the sesame seeds during a dry pan. Leave the sesame seeds to cool before Combining the dough.

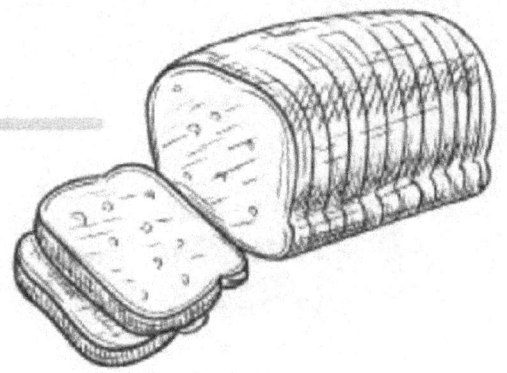

- When the dough is prepared, fastidiously kind into spherical loaves. After the loaves have risen for thirty minutes, flour and gently build incisions on high of the loaves before inserting them in the oven.

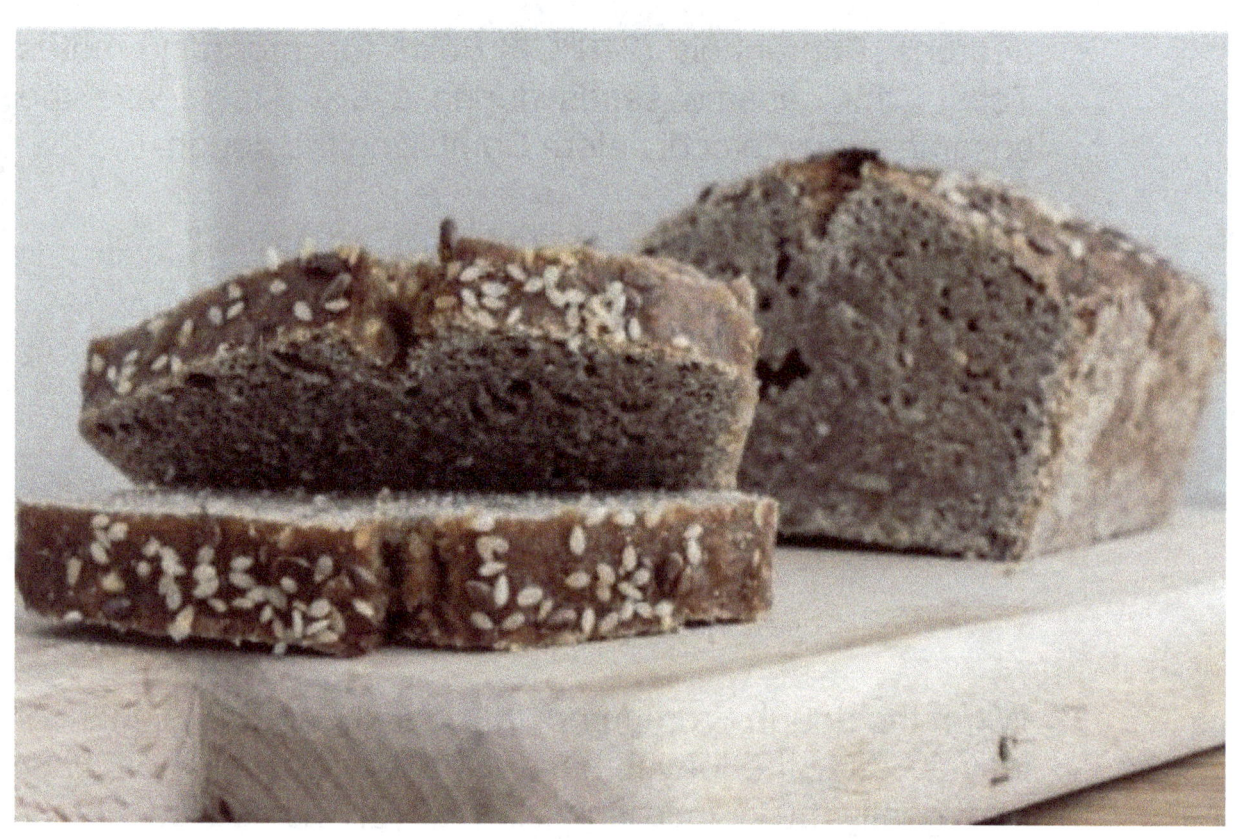

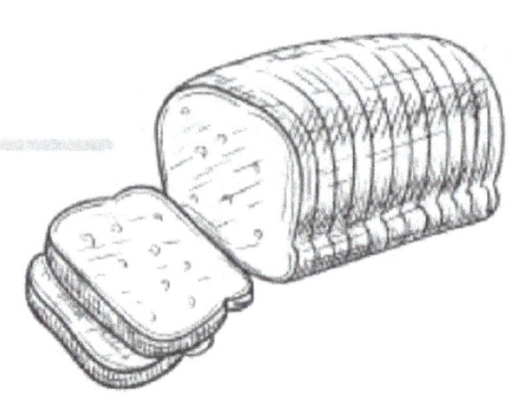

Wheat Malted Sourdough

Ingredients:

- 1 mug whole wheat Flour – 4.2 – Ounce
- half mug cracked Malted Rye Berries
- 1 mug vigorous Deem starter – 9 Ounce at 100% hydration
- 2 half mugs water – 20 Ounce
- 2 mugs rye Flour – 7.2 Ounce
- half mug regular cracked wheat – 2.7 Ounce

Instructions:

- Consolidate all fixings with the exception excepted and afterward empower the mixture to rest for twenty minutes (batter autolysis). At the point when autolysis, add salt and afterward Combine mixture on low speed for with concerning minutes. Mass mature (introductory ascent) for 4 - half-inebriated hours till mix the has multiplied. At the point when mass maturation, pour the batter onto a softly floured (Rye flour) sure and massage enough to accumulate into a ball.
- Gap the mixture and shape into the general shape you need and afterward empower the batter to rest for five – 10 minutes (seat rest). Next structure portions into their last shapes and put them into the lined or floured sealing bushels, container, or Couche. Empower the mixture to definite evidence for in regards to a couple of hours (till almost multiplied anyway delicate when you press in a finger).
- At that point cut, splash, and prepare, on top of a heating stone, during a preheated 450F/232.2C degree stove for twenty minutes

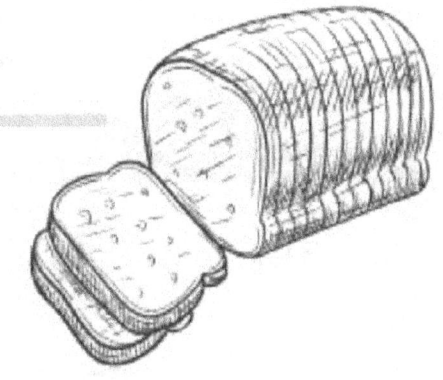

utilizing the Roasting Pan Method for steaming. After the initial 20 minutes, flip the stove down to 400F/204.4C degrees and keep preparing for in regards to 15 - 20 additional minutes or until your bread.

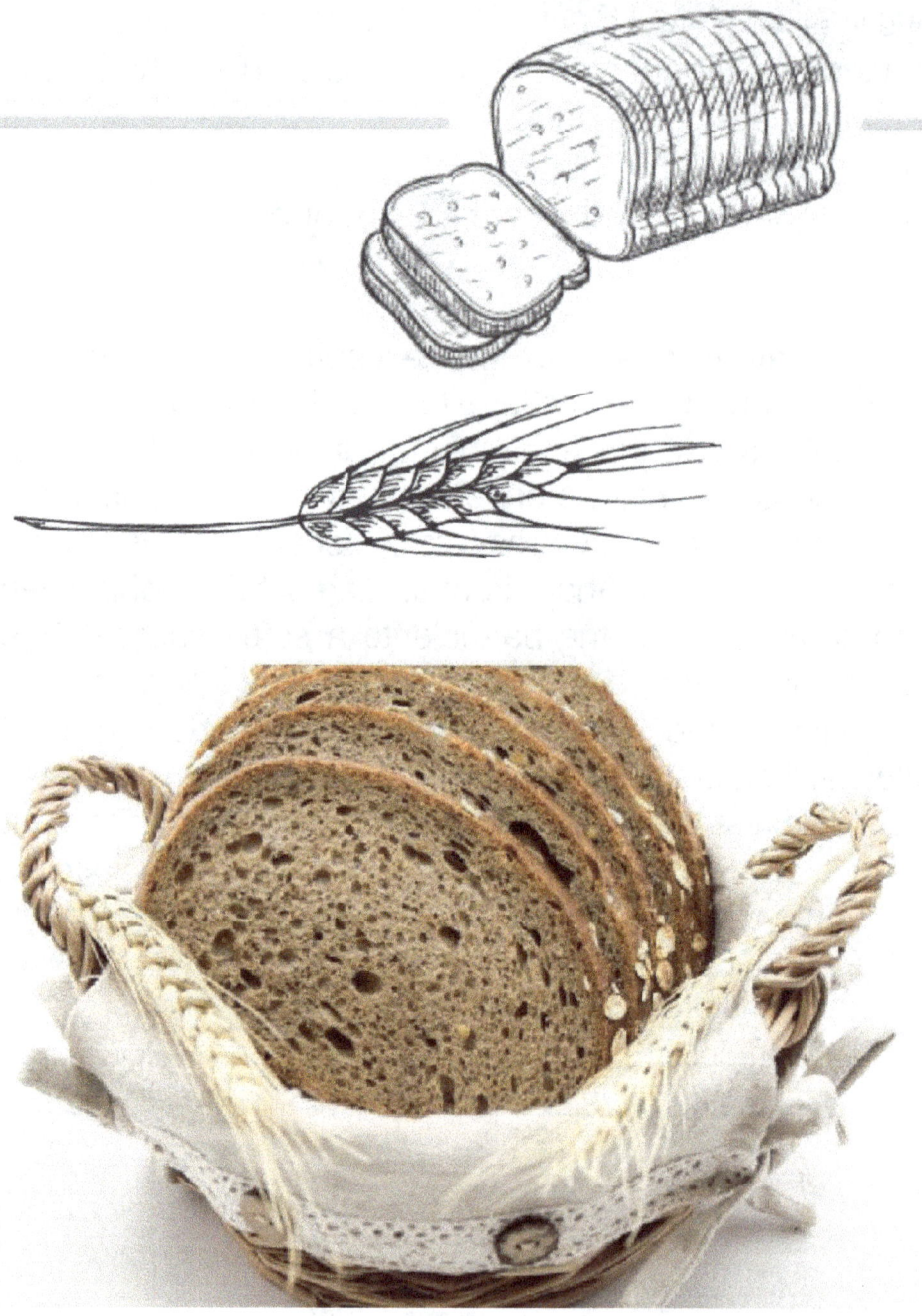

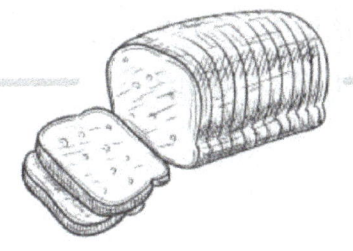

White Sourdough Bread

Ingredients:

- half mug (50 g) uncombined rye flour (i.e., flour without wheat)
- mugs (450 ml) water, room temperature
- 6 mugs (750 g) wheat flour
- 3half Ounce (100 g) wheat sourdough
- starter 1 mug (200 ml) water, room
- temperature 1one-fourth mug (150 g)
- wheat flour tsp (20 g) sea salt

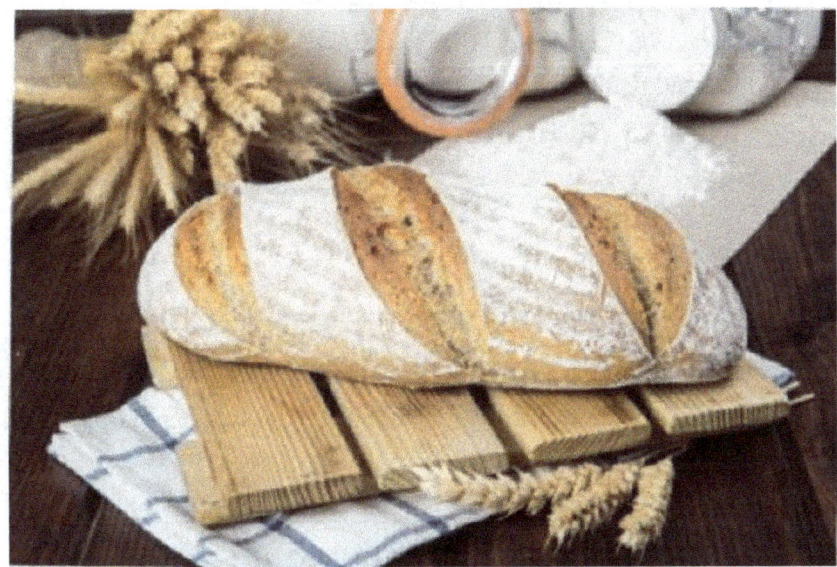

Instructions:

- Mix the flour and water into the dough. Knead the dough thoroughly. Toss in a pinch of salt. Knead the dough for another 2 minutes. Allow an hour for the dough to rise before forming into two loaves.
- Allow 45 minutes for the loaves to grow under a cloth. At the start, the oven temperature was 525 degrees Fahrenheit (280 degrees Celsius). Preheat the oven to 350 degrees. Preheat the

oven to 350°F. Place the loaves in the oven. Fill the bottom of the oven with a mug of water.

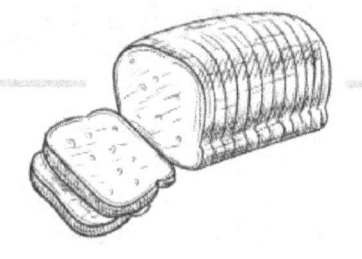

Asian Sourdough Bread

Ingredients:

- Ounce (150 g) wheat sourdough starter
- 1 tbsp (15 g) salt
- 1 tbsp raw sugar
- third-fourth Ounce (20 g) fresh yeast 1one-
- fourth mug (300 ml) water, room temperature
- 5half mugs (650 g) whole wheat flour one-
- fourth mug (50 ml) olive oil melted butter for
- brushing

Instructions:

- In a small amount of water, dissolve the yeast. Combine all of the ingredients in a large Combining bowl and knead thoroughly. Try adding a little at a time if you need more water than what is listed.
- Since the flour's responsiveness varies, the number is just an estimate. Form the kneaded dough into a loaf and let it rise for 45–60 minutes, or until it has doubled in length .

Yeast Sourdough

Ingredients:

- half mug (100 ml) water, room
- temperature 6 mugs (625 g) fine rye flour
- 1third-fourth mug (225 g) wheat flour

- 35 Ounce (1 kg) spelled sourdough starter
- 1 tbsp (15 g) salt
- tbsp (25 g) fresh yeast
- 2half tbsp (35 ml) treacle syrup (can be substituted with dark syrup)

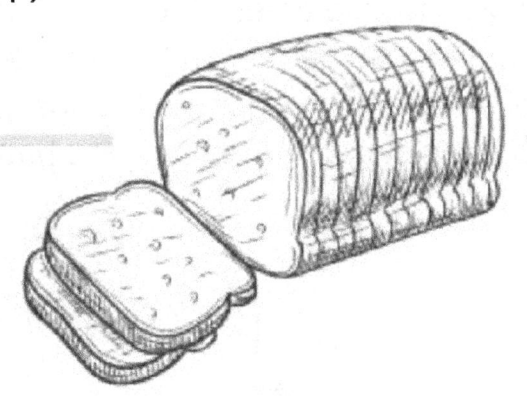

Instructions:

- After thoroughly mixing the ingredients, allow for a 30-minute increase. Flour the dough and gently shape it into two oblong loaves.
- Allow the bread to rise until it is twice its original size (let them rise in a basket, if possible). Preheat the oven to 475 degrees Fahrenheit (250 degrees Celsius). Place the loaves in the oven and use a mug of water to brush the oven surface.

Eastern Wheat Sourdough
Ingredients:

- 1 Tablespoon dark Molasses - .7
- Ounce 1/3 mug rye flour – 1.8 Ounce
- 2 1/3 mugs Whole Wheat flour – 9.7 Ounce
- 4 half mugs Bread flour –1 pound 4.3 Ounce
- 2 mug vigorous sourdough starter –18
- Ounce 1third-fourth mugs water tepid water–
- 14 Ounce half mug dry milk – .8 Ounce
- 2 TBSP oil –1 Ounce
- 1 Tablespoon malt syrup - .8 Ounce
- 3 half tsp salt - .7 Ounce (add after dough autolysis)

Instructions:

- After autolysis, add salt and consolidate batter on low speed for a couple of minutes. At that point let the batter mass mature for 6-8 hours. Mix the batter down with only three turns of the mixture snare multiple times all through the vi - eight-hour mass maturation or crease batter in a battered box.
- This is to reinforce the gluten strands and line them up, in addition to it assists with remaining the batter from over aging. After mass maturation, pour the mixture onto a gently floured (Whole Wheat flour) surface and work a couple of times at that point accumulate into a ball. Gap the batter into 2 pieces.
- Structure portions into the last structure you need and afterward empower the batter to rest for five-ten minutes (seat rest). After sidelining shape portions into their last shapes and put them into the sealing containers (Bannetons don't should be lined). Empower the batter to line out for half-hour and afterward refrigerate for the time being.
- You will skirt the half-hour stand by if the batter has been extremely enthusiastic for the day. Next morning dispose of the portions staggered thirty minutes separated (hence you don't ought to prepare them simultaneously) at that point permit the batter to ascend until sealing is finished. This can take somewhere in the range of 1 - three hours and is the point at which the batter will increment in size concerning 1 half times.

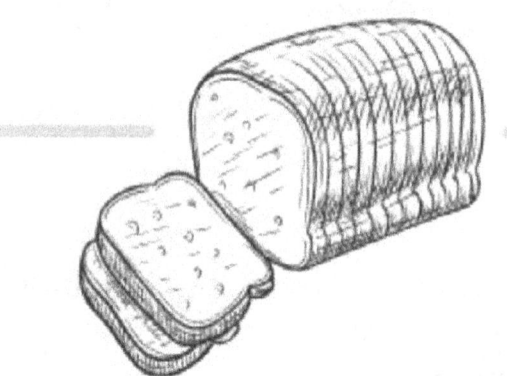

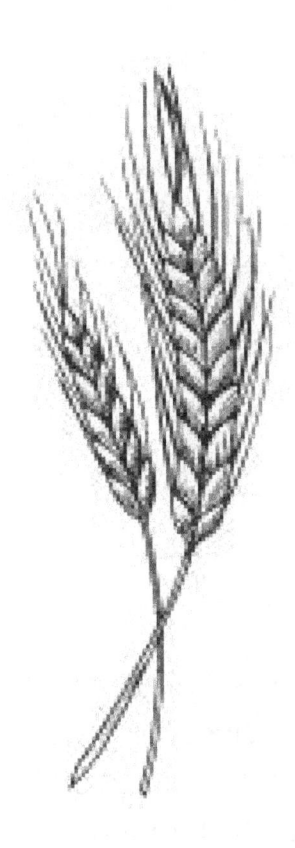

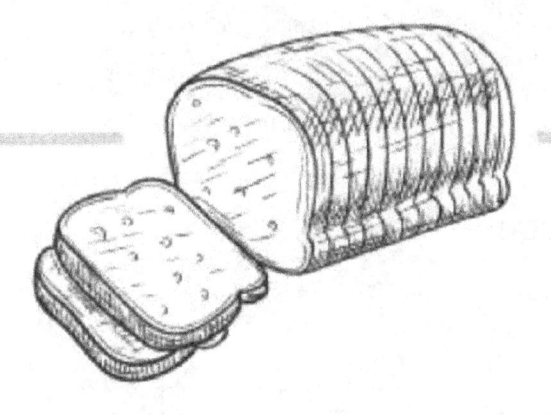

Carrot Milky Sourdough

Ingredients:

- 1 mug (100 g) rolled oats (dry roast them in a non-stick frying pan)
- Ounce (150 g) wheat sourdough
- starter 1 mug (200 ml) water, room
- temperature half mug (100 ml) milk,
- room temperature 1third-fourth tsp (5
- g) fresh yeast 1 tbsp (15 g) salt
- 3third-fourth mugs (450 g) wheat flour,
- wholemeal mugs wholemeal and carrots

Instructions:

- Combine the milk and yeast. Combine all ingredients, aside from the carrots. Knead the dough for concerning ten minutes. Add the grated carrots and knead some additional. Let the dough rise for 60-90 minutes during a warm place.
- Note that the dough can be slightly sticky. When the dough has risen fully, it ought to be kneaded once more. Fill 2 to 3 greased pans halfway with dough.

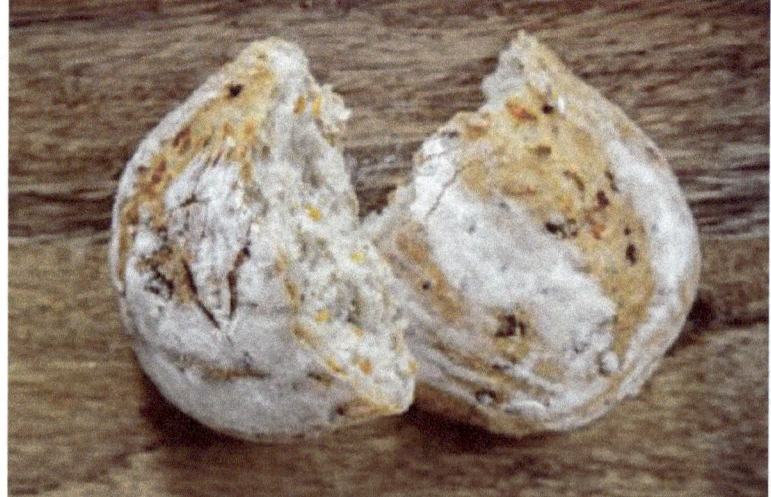

Let the dough rise for 45 mutual times vary slightly-the dough is prepared when it's doubled in size. Initial Oven Temperature:

475degrees

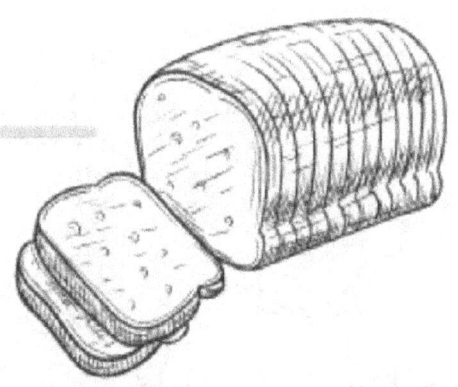

Fahrenheit(250°C) Place the loaves within the oven and bake for 10 minutes.

- Lower the temperature to 350degrees Fahrenheit(180°C) and bake for roughly thirty minutes additional. Roast the oats in a very non-stick frying pan. Knead the dough for regarding tended the grated carrot. Fill the pans halfway with the fermented and loose dough.

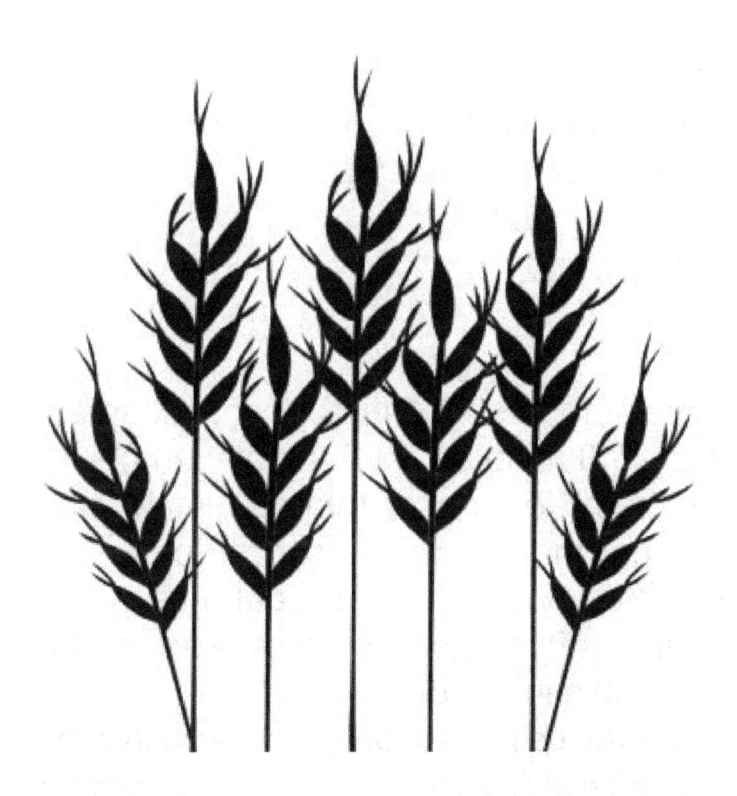

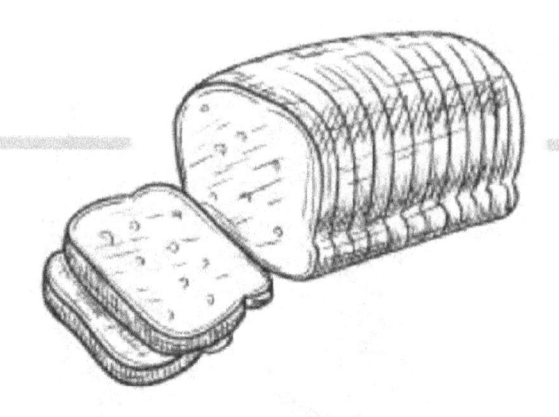

Dark Beer Rye Sourdough

Ingredients:

- 1 Tablespoon Dark Molasses - .7 Ounce/19.8g
- 3 Tbsp dried toasted onion flakes - .6 Ounce/17g
- 3 Tbsp Caraway seeds – 1 Ounce/28g
- 3 mugs Bread flour -13.5 Ounce/382g
- 2 mugs Rye starter at 100% hydration – 18 Ounce/510g
- 1 mug water – 6Ounce/170g
- 1 dark rich beer – 12 Ounce/340g
- 3 Tbsp Oil – 1.5 Ounce/42g
- 1 Tablespoon non-diastatic malt syrup -.8 Ounce/2malt mugs Whole Wheat flour – 12.6 Ounce/357g
- 2 mugs Rye flour – 7.2 Ounce/204g
- 4 tsp of Sea Salt - .8 Ounce/22.7g

Instructions:

- Join the fixings on a medium speed simply till consolidated, this takes in regards to 2 - 3 minutes. At that point empower the batter to autolyze (rest) for twenty minutes. mass age (which simply implies that the essential ascent) for 4 - six hours until multiplied. After massaging, spill out massaging onto a delicately floured (Rye flour) surface and a few times, at that point assemble into a ball.
- Gap the batter into two enormous pieces. Shape portions into the last shape you need and afterward permit the mixture to rest for five minutes (seat rest). After side After structure portions into their last shapes and put them into the sealing bushels, or

containers that are fixed with sealing fabrics on the off chance that you need (Bannetons don't should be lined). Refrigerate for the time being. Next morning,

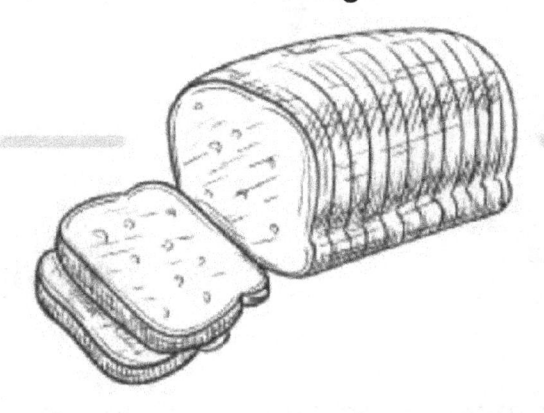

cast off the mixture staggered concerning 40 microns concerning granting the batter to warm up and verification this ought to be the point at which the batter increments in volume one a large portion of the measurements.

- You must be extra mindful so as not to overproof Rye bread at the point when the mixture is prepared and feels effervescent and springy yet not droopy, at that point taking the main portion sprinkle the prime (actually the underside) with semolina or the entire grain flour and flip the batter out onto a strip of level heating sheet. At that point slice the batter while still on the strip, slide into the hot preheated 450F/232.2C degree stove onto a hot preparing stone, shower the mixture once with water rapidly, and afterward cover with a simmering top which has also been preheated in the broiler. Heat for twenty minutes. After 20minutes, start the cooking top and turn down the broiler to 400F/204.4C degrees. Keep preparing for 18 - 25 a ton of minutes, or until your bread thermometer peruses 200 205F/93-96C.
- Flip the portion partially through the last preparing period for searing. Cool. For the resulting portion, turn the broiler keep a duplicate, and set the simmering cover back in to preheat for 5 - ten minutes or until the portion is set up to go in. Heat the indistinguishable as the essential portion. Cool this heavenly bread and eat with late spread and cream cheddar. This bread

incorporates a dull, harsh, delectable flavor, and is pleasant for sandwiches.

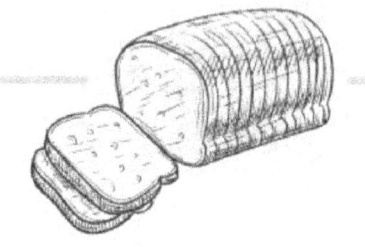

Mexican Sourdough

Ingredients:

- half mug mashed potatoes – 4 Ounce
- 6 2/3 mugs of Bread flour – 1Poundd 14 Ounce
- 2 mugs sourdough starter – 18 Ounce at 166%
- hydration 1third-fourth mugs water – 14 Ounce
- 2 Tbsp of Oil – 1 Ounce
- 1 Tbsp malt syrup or honey – .8
- Ounce 2/3 mug Whole Wheat flour –
- 2 .8 Ounce 4 tsp of Salt – .8 Ounce

Instructions:

- Join the fixings on a medium speed just until consolidated, this requires around two minutes. At that point license the batter to autolyze (rest) for twenty minutes. After autolysis, consolidate batter on low speed for concerning 1 moment. At that point let the mixture mass mature (which implies that the main ascent) for 4 - half-tanked hours till multiplied. Flip the mixture down at least twice all through the lion's share age which creates and lines up the gluten strands.
- To attempt this hit the starting catcher and let the snare mix the batter concerning twice around the bowl on the absolute bottom setting. After mass maturation, pour the batter onto a daintily floured surface and work on various occasions, at that point assemble it into a ball. Separation the mixture into two pieces. Structure portions into the general shape you might want and afterward empower the mixture to rest for ten minutes (seat rest).

In the wake of sidelining, structure portions into their last shapes and spot them into lined sealing crates (Bannetons don't should be lined).

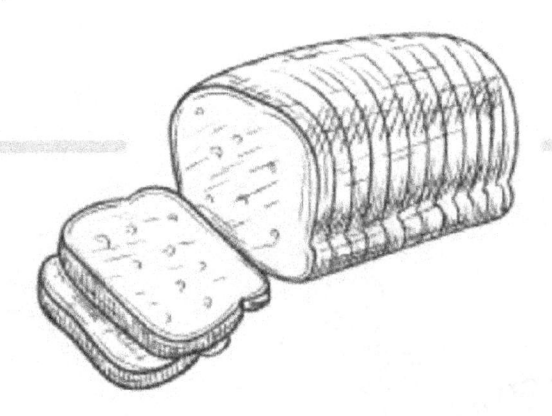

- Let mixture began for thirty minutes and afterward cowl the batter with plastic gear and refrigerate for the time being. Toward the beginning of the day, permit the batter to definite evidence for around two hours (mixture can look multiplied and supple/springy) and afterward flip the mixture out onto a strip and slice, splash, cowl with broiling cover and heat in an extremely preheated 450F/232C degree stove for twenty minutes. Following 20 minutes, remove the cooking top, flip down the broiler to 400F/204.4C degrees and keep preparing for concerning 10-15 a lot of minutes, turning most of the way for searing.

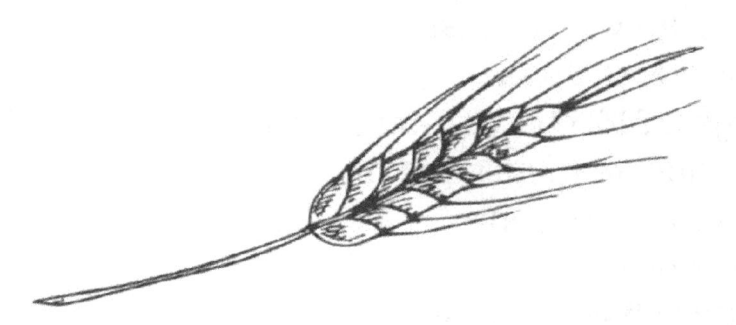

- Take out portion and out of control on a rack. On the off chance that your first portion turns out too earthy colored, flip the broiler directly down to 425F/218.3C degrees all through the essential 0.5 of the prepares as opposed to 450F/232C degrees. Remember to put the simmering top once more into the broiler and warm to 450 degrees once more, before placing it in the following portion. This might be a brilliant, scrumptious portion and is awesome with spread or utilized for sandwiches.

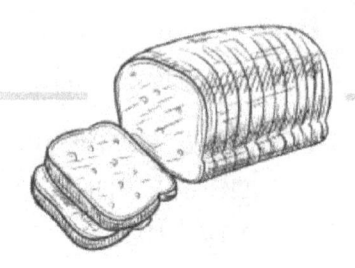

Cheddar Sourdough

Ingredients:

- 1 teaspoon kosher salt
- 2 tbsp unsalted butter
- 4 ounces shredded mild
- Cheddar
- 1 mug fresh corn kernels,
- mug room temperature water
- 2 1/4 tsp active dry yeast
- 1 tablespoon sugar
- 3 mugs (13 1/2 ounces) sourdough
- flour, plus more as needed
- roughly chopped into
- smaller pieces
- Nonstock baking spray

Instructions:

- Consolidate the water, yeast, sugar, flour, salt, and margarine and ply by hand (join first in an extremely enormous bowl, at that point flip out and massage) or in a stand mixer fitted with the mixture snare until smooth. The batter will be genuinely hardened now. Add the cheddar and corn and keep massaging just until they're joined. At introductory, the batter will appear to be wet and messy from the dampness inside the corn, but since the corn becomes fused, the mixture will get milder and firm.

- Cover the bowl and put aside to ascend until the mixture has multiplied in size, in regard to 1 hour in a very warm room. Splash a nine x 5-in. portion skillet with a preparing shower.

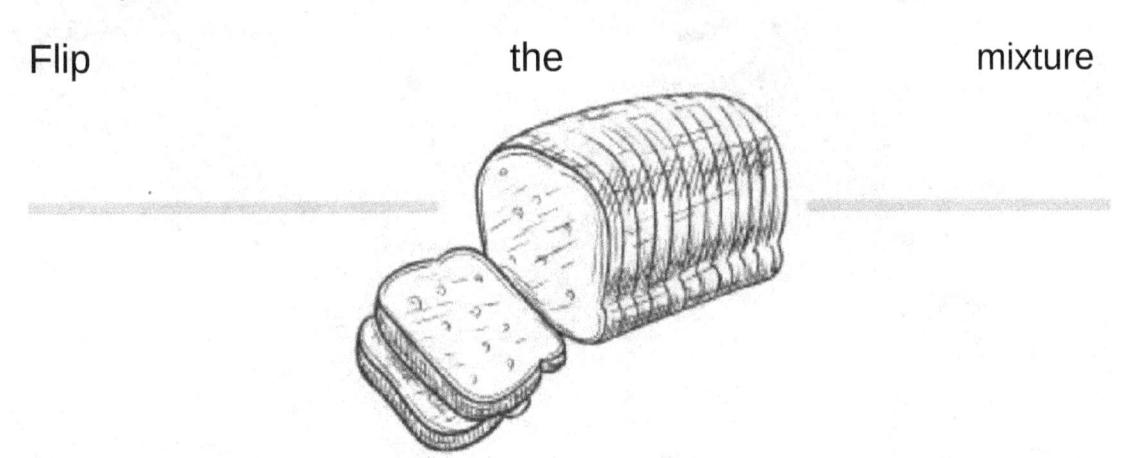

Flip the mixture out onto a daintily floured surface and pat it into a harsh 8-in. square. Overlap the prime to concerning the focal point of the batter and press the edge directly down to get it. Overlay the prime over again, this highlights inside about an in. or then again accordingly of the underside.

- Press the edge to seal. Presently pull the underside of the batter up to satisfy the mixture roll you've made and seal the crease. Squeeze the finishes shut and place the batter, crease feature down, in the readied portion dish. Cover the skillet with saran wrap or spot the full container during an enormous plastic sack and tie the open completion shut. Refrigerate for the time being or as long as 24 hours before preparing. The mixture should completely rise when around 6 hours.

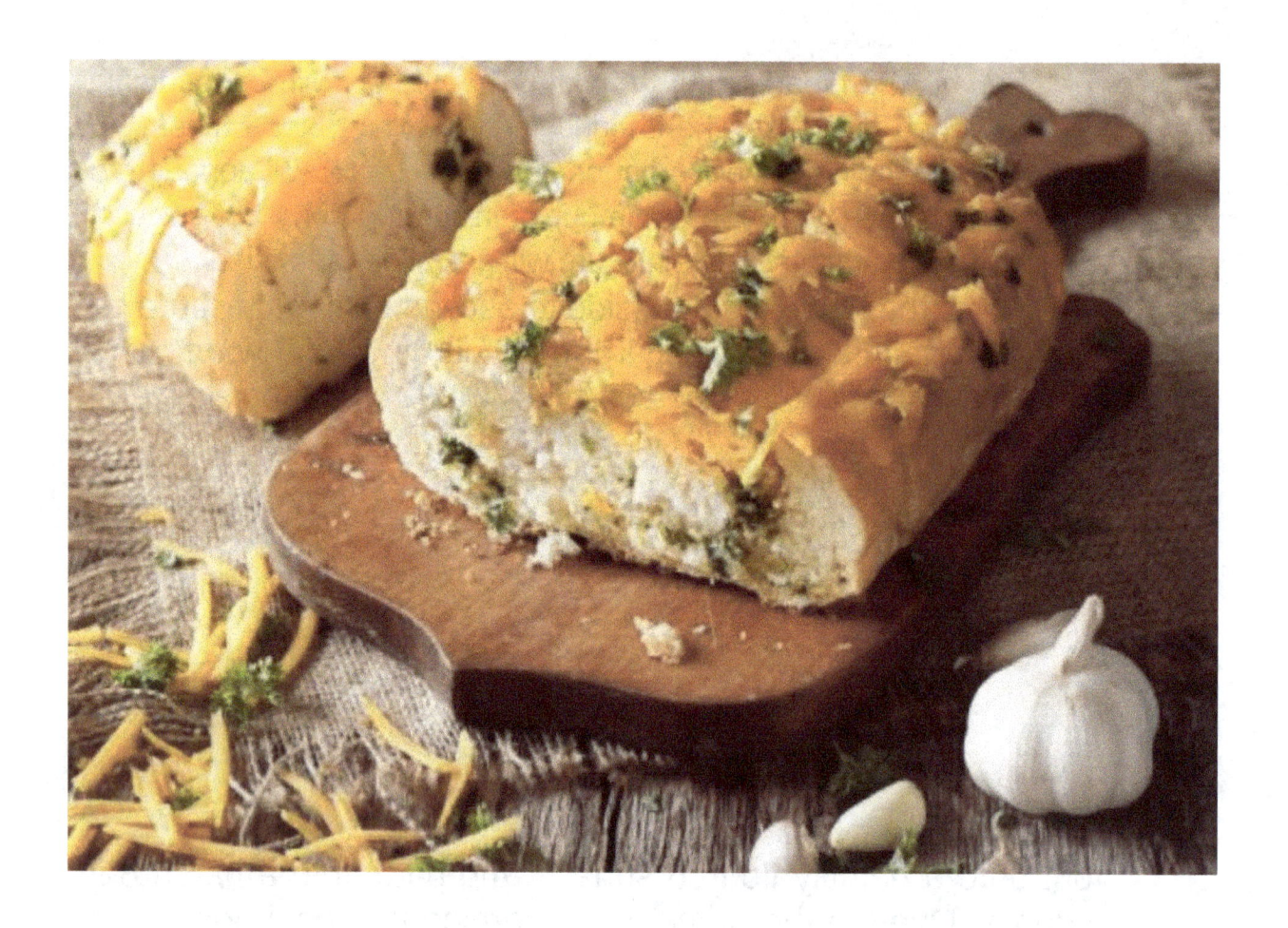

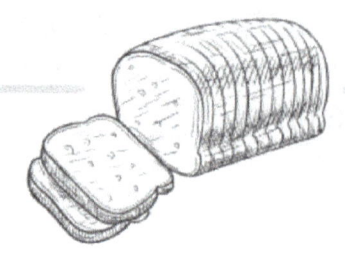

Danish Sourdough

Ingredients:

- 2 mugs Dark Rye Flour – 7.2 Ounce/204g

- 2 mugs Whole Wheat Flour – 8.4 Ounce/238g
- 3 mugs Bread Flour – 13.5 Ounce/382g
- 2 mugs vigorous Danish Rye starter at 100% hydration
- 2 mugs strong coffee – 16 Ounce/453g
- 3 Tbsp oil – 1.5 Ounce/42g
- 2 Tbsp Molasses – 1.4 Ounce/39.7g
- 3 half tsp salt – .7 Ounce/19.8g

Instructions:

- Consolidate all fixings together prepares with salt, just until joined, and afterward permit the batter to rest for twenty minutes (autolyze). After autolysis, join batter on low speed for about a couple of minutes. At that point let the mixture mass mature (first ascent) for six hours. When mass maturation, spill out the mixture onto a tenderly floured (Rye flour) surface and ply enough to amass into a ball.
- Separation the batter. I separated the mixture into 2 goliath portions gauging a little over a couple of pounds. each. Shape mixture into the general shape you might want and afterward permit the batter to rest for five - 10 minutes (seat rest). While sidelining, shape portions into their last shapes and put them into the sealing containers, skillet, or Couche. Spot bannetons in plastic baggage and refrigerate for the time being. Toward the beginning of the day, license the mixture to conclusive evidence for 2 - 2.5 hours (till essentially multiplied anyway delicate once you press during a finger) at that point slice,

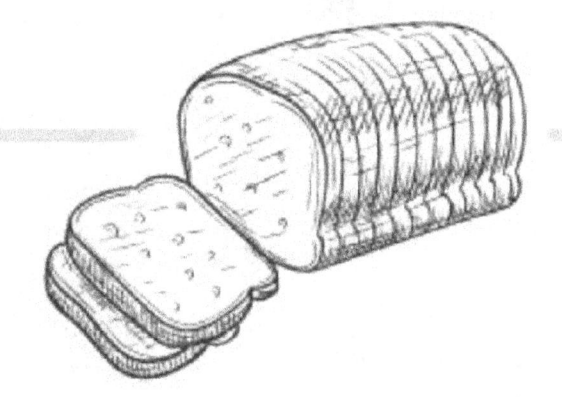

shower, and prepare, on top of a heating stone, in a preheated

450F/232.2C degree stove for twenty minutes utilizing the Roasting Pan Method for steaming.

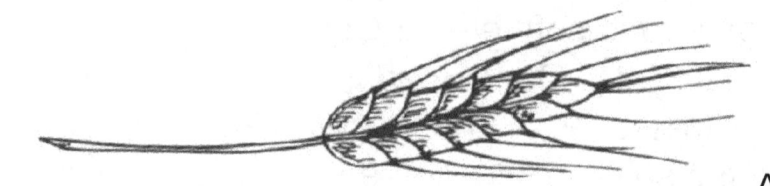

- After the essential twenty minutes, turn down the broiler to 400F/204.4C degrees and keep heating for concerning eighteen - 25 additional minutes, or till your bread thermometer peruses 200 205F/93 96C, turning most of the way for cooking. Cool. This might be a tasty, vigorous enhanced rye and freezes well.

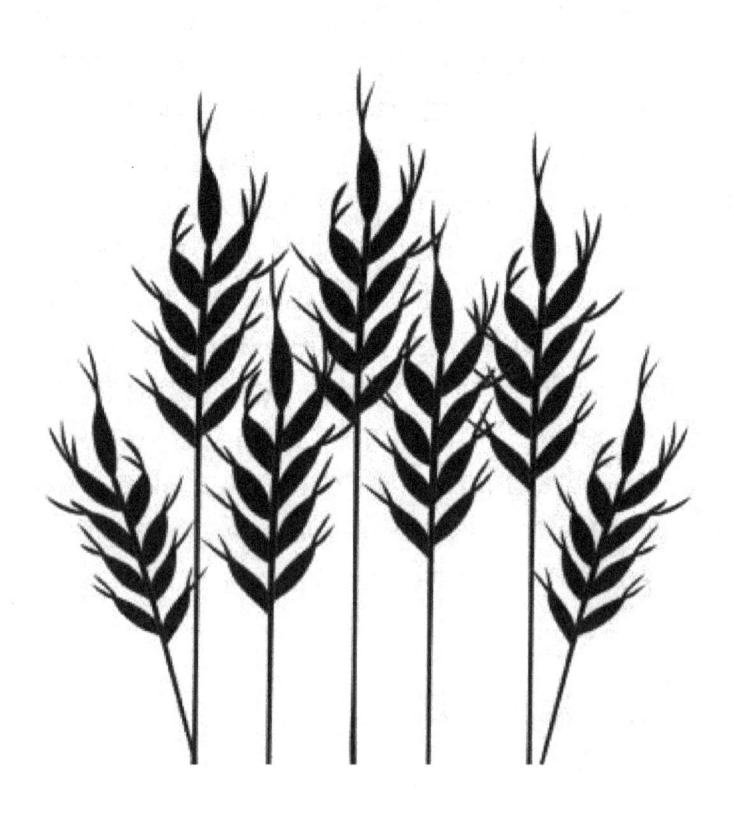

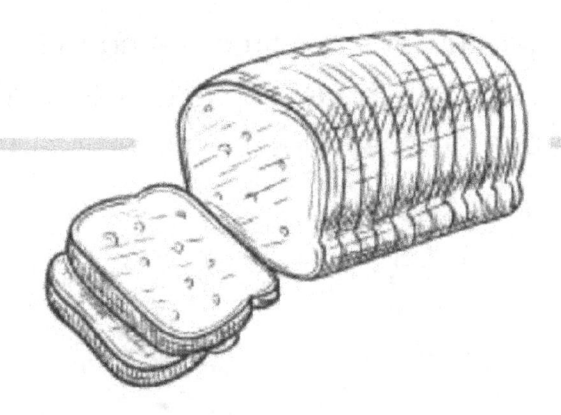

Milky Grain Sourdough

Ingredients:

- 1 Tablespoon Millet seeds - .4 Ounce
- one-fourth mug flax seeds – 1.5 Ounce
- 1 mug boiling water – 8 Ounce
- 1 mug of Combined cracked wheat and rye – 6 Ounce
- 1 Tablespoon Malt syrup - .8 Ounce
- 1 Tablespoon Sesame or Dill seeds -.4 Ounce one-fourth
- mug sunflower seeds or Combined seeds/trail Combine – 1.5 Ounce

Instructions:

- On the off chance that you added more than the suggested seeds, you'll need to highlight extra water or less flour to make up contrast inside the fluid sum required. Interaction this

inside the Mixer for 2 to a couple of moments at that point let the mixture one-half autolysis for twenty minutes. Next, add the cooled seed/grain Mixture and accordingly the salt to the batter and Combine in well. Permit the mixture to mass mature for concerning 6 hours. During the massage, crease the mixture like clockwork.

- At the point when mass mature is done, push down the batter and move it to a delicately floured surface utilizing rye flour. Work the batter barely enough to collect it into a ball. Separation the batter into two things and shape the portions of bread. Spot mixture into floured or lined bushels, cover with a plastic pack, and refrigerate for the time being. Next morning, remove portions from the fridge (amaze the portions concerning 30 minutes separated) and let the mixture warm-up and evidence.

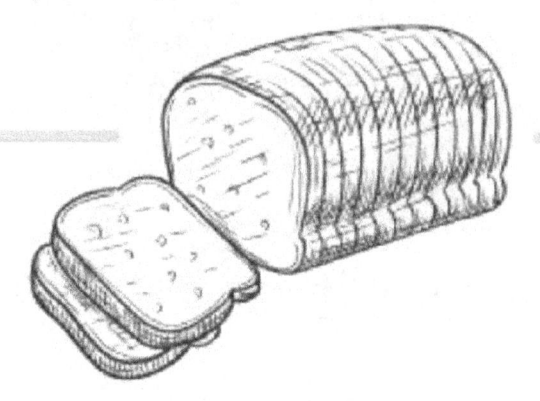

- Since this bread is loaded up with seeds; it can take the mixture longer to evidence (anticipate that it should take a couple of-three hours or extra). At the point when the mixture is arranged and feels effervescent and springy however not droopy at, that point, taking the main portion sprinkle the top (really the base) with semolina or rye flour and turn the batter out onto a strip of level heating sheet.

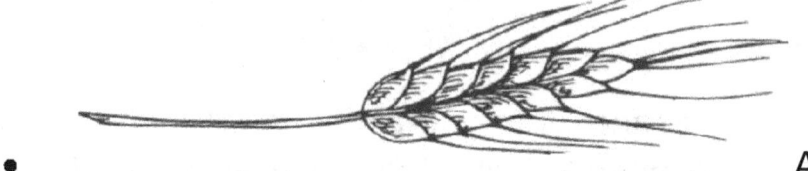

- At that point cut the mixture while still on the strip, slide into the new preheated 450F/232C degree stove onto a hot heating stone, splash the batter once with water rapidly, and afterward cowl with a broiling cover that has also been preheated inside the broiler.

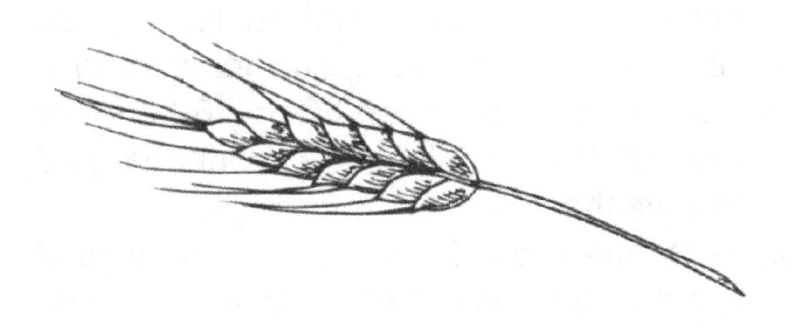

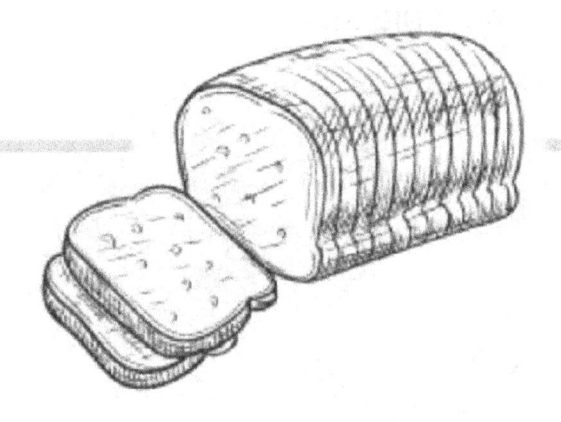

Spicy Jalapeno Sourdough

Ingredients:

- half mug Rye flour – 1.8 Ounce
- 2 mugs Bread flour – 9 Ounce
- 1 mug vigorous sourdough starter at 166% hydration -9Ounce
- 1 half mugs water – 12 Ounce
- half mug Whole Wheat flour – 2.1 Ounce

Instructions:

- Join all fixings, including salt together and let rest for 20 minutes. At that point strategy on low speed for around 4 extra minutes. Let confirmation for around four - 6 hours or multiplied. Have around 8 Ounce Jalapeno cheddar lumped for each portion. Separate the batter into two things.
- Take one piece of the mixture and unfurl it out into a rectangular structure, press in regard to four Ounces of the lumped cheddar into the batter, at that point overlay the batter into thirds. Smooth the batter out, press on the contrary 4 Ounces of cheddar, and crease into thirds again. At that point let the mixture rest five minutes and end forming into your portion by collapsing over and squeezing the batter at the base. Spot the batter into a lubed bread skillet or spot in a banneton/crate.
- Structure different portions and afterward let confirmation for two-three hours or till the batter increments in size concerning 1 half time.
- Then slice the batter though still on the strip, slide into the new preheated 400F/204.2C degree stove onto a hot heating stone, splash

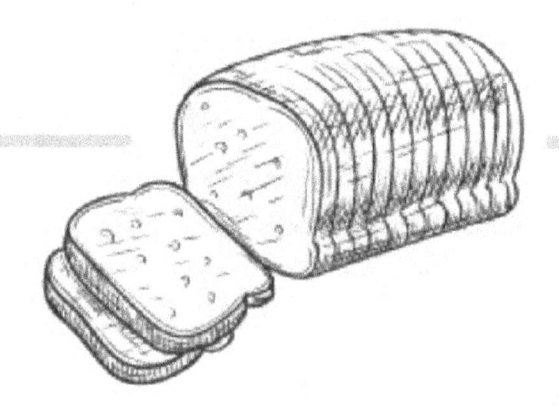

the mixture once with water rapidly, and afterward cowl with a simmering top that has additionally been preheated inside the broiler.

- Prepare for twenty minutes. After 20minutes, set out the broiling cover and keep preparing for 15 – twenty a lot of minutes or until your bread thermometer peruses 200-205F/93-96C. Turn the portion partially through the last preparing period for cooking. Cool. For the following portion, flip the broiler keep a duplicate and spot the simmering top back in to preheat for 5 - 10 minutes or till the portion is prepared to go in.

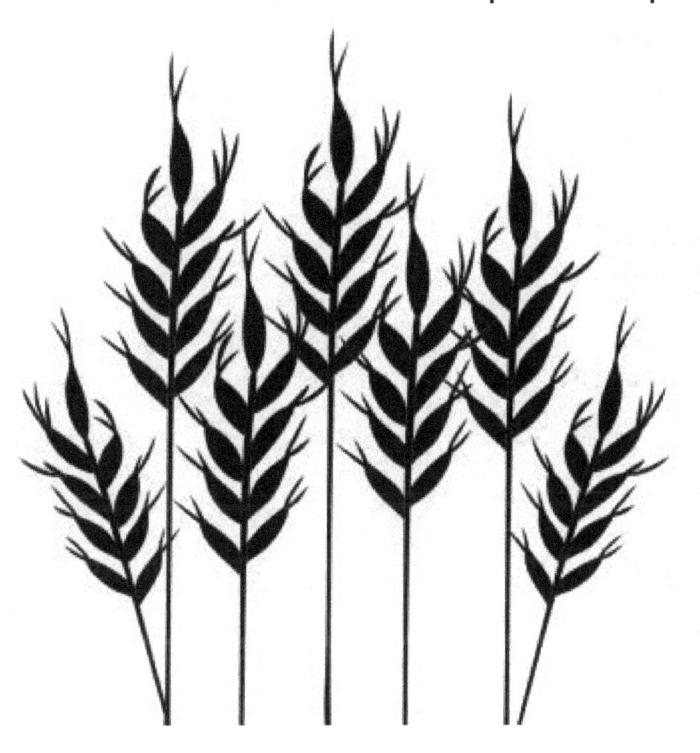

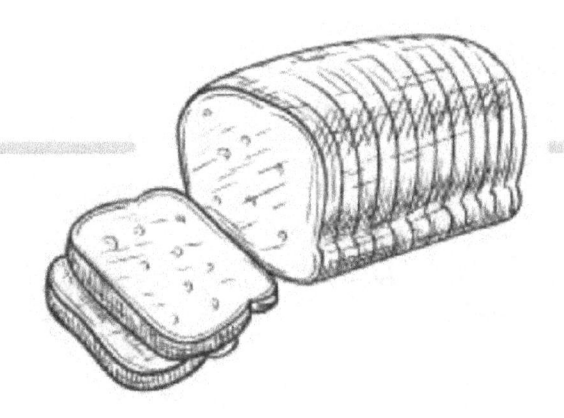

White, Whole Wheat Sourdough

Ingredients:

- sourdough flour
- 1/2 mug (2 1/2 ounces) dark
- rye flour
- 1/2 teaspoon kosher salt
- 1 teaspoon vital wheat gluten
- 1 teaspoon cocoa powder
- 1/2 mug plus 1 tablespoon room
- temperature water
- 1 teaspoon active dry yeast
- 1 teaspoon sugar
- 3/4 mug (3 3/8 ounces)
- wheat flour
- 1/2 teaspoon kosher salt
- 1 teaspoon unsalted butter,
- at room temperature

Instructions:

- For every one of the three batters, the directions are the equivalent: Combine all fixings until joined (in a medium bowl or the bowl of your stand Mixer), at that point massage by hand or in a stand mixer fitted with the mixture snare until the mixture is versatile. I propose beginning with the rye batter, the wheat, at that point the white. (The rye rises a touch all the more gradually, so it's acceptable to give it

a head start; white ascents most rapidly.) After every batter is readied, place it in a medium bowl, cover it, and put it aside in a warm spot.

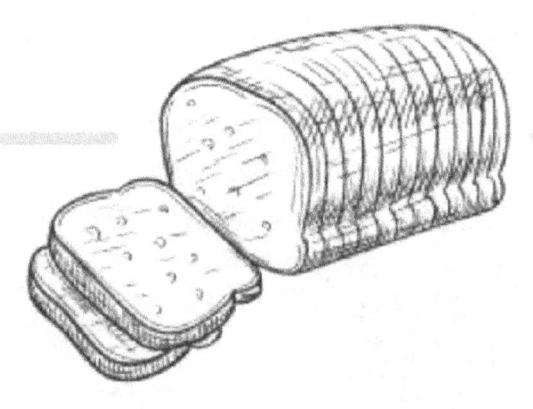

- At the point when you've wrapped up setting up the third mixture, set a clock for 45 minutes and let the entirety of the batters rise. Line a heating sheet with material paper. At the point when the batters have risen, flour your work surface daintily. Each, in turn, transform out every mixture and structure it into a rope (as a kid would roll a snake from dirt) around 20 inches in length. Line up the three bits of mixture close to one another. Squeeze the three together toward one side, at that point interlace them freely.

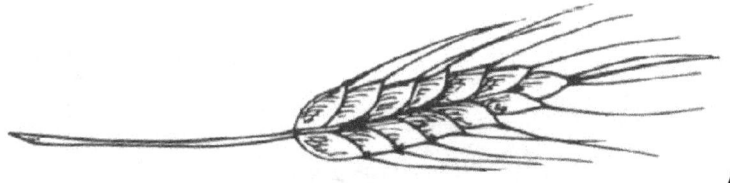

- At the point when you finish, squeeze the closures together. Move the batter to the material-lined preparing sheet. I like to organize it askew on the sheet for more space. Fold the squeezed finishes under to conceal them, and fix and mastermind the batter so it's even. Cover with cling wrap and refrigerate for the time being or as long as 24 hours.

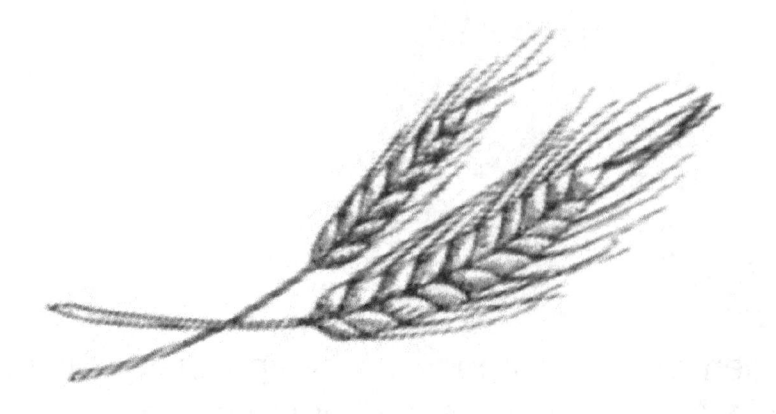

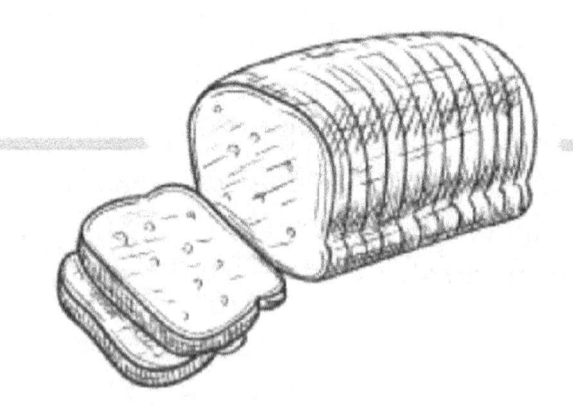

Garlic Onion Sourdough
Ingredients:

- 2 Tbsp Oil – 1 Ounce
- 1 teaspoon cracked black pepper -.07 Ounce
- 1 Tbsp Dill Seed -.23 Ounce
- Preferment

- Molasses
- Granulated Onion
- Powder
- 1 mug evaporated milk – 8 Ounce
- 1 Tbsp flaked red pepper -.08 Ounce

Instructions:

- Add five one-fourth mugs bread flour 4 tsp salt-.8 osmics the fixings remembering salt for medium speed just until consolidated, this takes around 2 - three minutes. The mixture will be tacky. At that point empower the mixture autolysis (rest) for 20 minutes. After autolysis, join batter on low speed for concerning four minutes. At that point let the mixture mass mature for in regards to 4 hours till multiplied. After massaging, pour the mixture onto a tenderly floured (Rye flour) surface and ply a couple of times, at that point accumulate into a ball. Separation the batter into 2 gigantic pieces. Structure portions into the overall structure you need and afterward license the mixture to rest for ten minutes (seat rest). After sidelining structure portions into their last shapes and put them into the sealing bins, or skillet that is

fixed with sealing materials on the off chance that you might want (Bannetons don't ought to be lined).

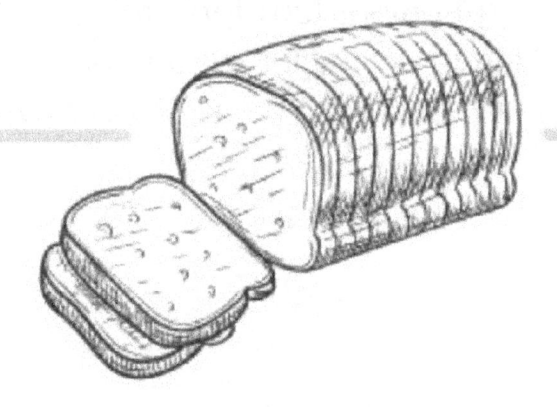

- Cowl the portions with fabrics and splash gently with water to keep the mixture damp, or put batter, bannetons, and each one into plastic packs. Grant mixture to evidence 1-3 hours or till arranged. You should keep an eye out not to overproof Rye bread. Preheat stove to 450F/232.2C degrees. At the point when the mixture is arranged and feels effervescent and springy yet not droopy, at that point taking the essential portion sprinkle the high (really the underside) with semolina or entire grain flour and flip the batter out onto a strip of level preparing sheet. At the point when arranged to prepare, turn your batter out onto a strip. At that point slice the batter while still on the strip, slide into the hot preheated 450F/232.2C degree stove onto a hot preparing stone, splash the mixture once with water rapidly, and afterward cowl with a simmering top which has furthermore been preheated in the broiler. Prepare for twenty minutes.

- After 20minutes, fire up the simmering cover and turn down the stove to 400F/204.4C degrees. Keep heating for 18 - 25 extra minutes or until your bread thermometer peruses 200 205F/93-96C. Flip the portion partially through the last heating sum for searing. Cool.

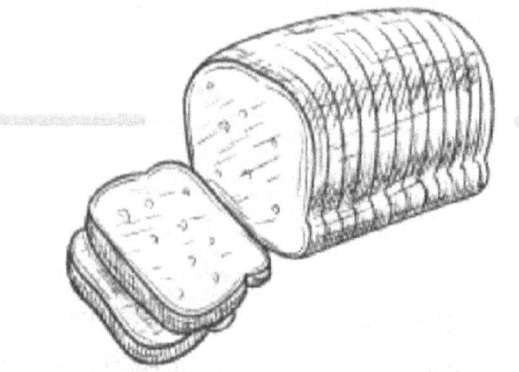

For the ensuing portion, turn the broiler make a duplicate, and spot the cooking cover back in to preheat for five - 10 minutes or till the portion is prepared to go in. Heat the indistinguishable as the essential portion. Cool this delightful bread and eat with a new spread and cream cheddar. This bread envelops a dim, made garlicky, onion flavor and is pleasant for store meat sandwiches.

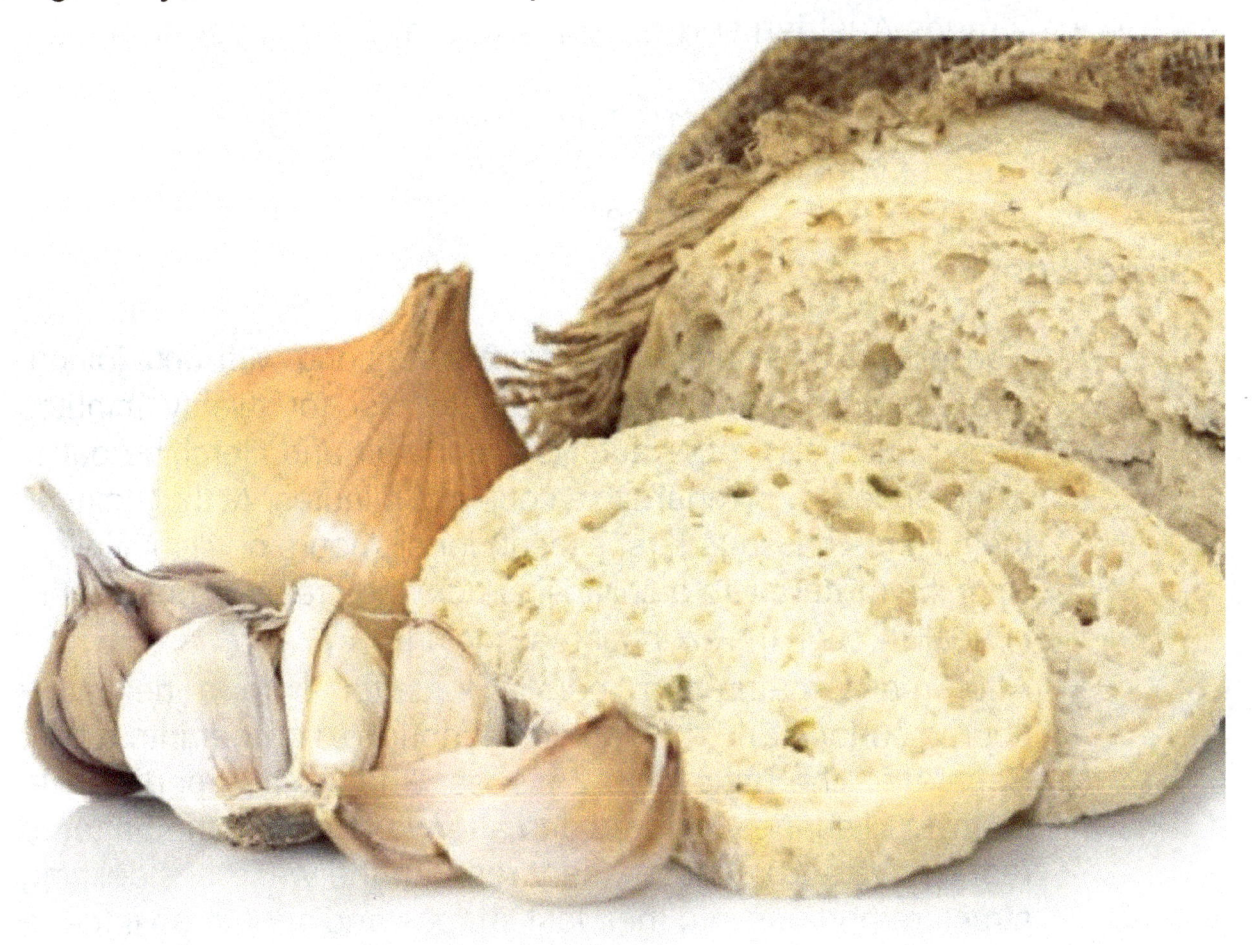

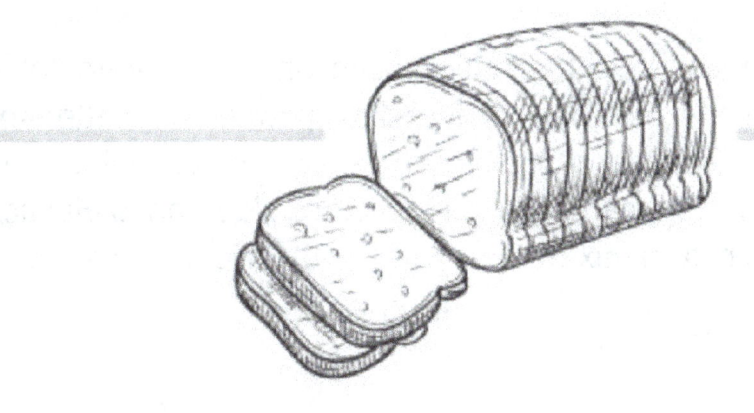

Modern Salty Sourdough
Ingredients:

- 1/3 mug rye flour -1.2 Ounce

- 8 2/3 mugs Bread Flour – 28.1 Ounce
- 2 mugs Austrian sourdough starter at 166% hydration – 18 Ounce
- 1 half mugs water – 12 Ounce third
- -fourth evaporated milk – 6 Ounce
- 4 half tsp salt – .9 Ounce

Instructions:

- Consolidate all fixings, aside from salt, along with until joined, and afterward permit the mixture to rest for twenty minutes (batter autolysis). After autolysis, add salt and Combine batter at low speed for in regard to a couple of minutes. At that point let the mixture massage (first ascent) for six hours or till multiplied. Spot the mixture into a collapsing box and crease it once every hour all through the six-hour massaging.
- After mass maturation, pour the batter onto a delicately floured surface and manipulate it enough to gather into a ball. Separation the batter into 2 pieces. Shape each portion into the overall shape you need and afterward license the batter to rest for five – 10 minutes (seat rest). In the wake of sidelining structure portions into their last shapes and spot them into the sealing crates, dish, or Couche.
- Cowl the batter with plastic sacks and refrigerate for the time being. In the first part of the day, permit the batter to definite evidence for 2 – three hours (at whatever point the mixture appearance concerning 1 half times its size and is elastic/springy) at that point turn mixture out on strip and slice, shower, cowl with simmering top

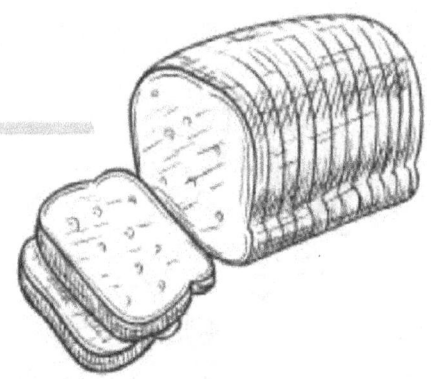

and prepare during a preheated 425F/218C degree stove for 20 minutes. Following 20 minutes, remove the simmering cover, flip down the stove to 400F/204C degrees and keep preparing for around ten-15 extra minutes, turning most of the way for caramelizing.
- Bread is finished when the inside temperature arrives at 200-205F/93 96C. Take out portion and cool on a rack. If your underlying portion appears to be excessively earthy colored, keep the temperature of the stove at 425F/218C degrees all through the entire heating period on the accompanying prepare. Remember to return the broiling cover to the stove to preheat before placing it in the resulting portion.

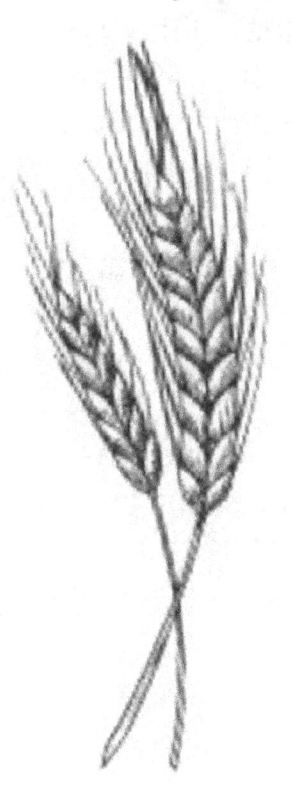

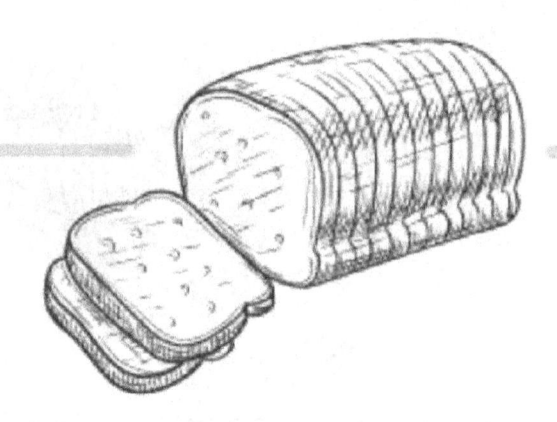

Buckwheat Delicious Sourdough

Ingredients:

- 1 mug Whole Wheat flour – 4.2 Ounce
- 1 mug of sourdough starter at 166% hydration -9 Ounce
- 2 mugs of water-16 Ounce
- 1 Mug coarsely ground Buckwheat -4.6 Ounce
- 2 mugs bread flour- 9 Ounce

Instructions:

- Consolidate the fixings, except the salt, along till all-around joined (concerning a couple of – three minutes) at that point let the batter rest for 20 minutes (mixture autolysis). After mixture autolysis, add the salt and consolidate the batter on low speed for four minutes more. Allow this batter to verification for concerning four hours or till multiplied in size. At that point shape the portions, amazing molding 30 minutes separated.
- Allow the mixture to heat up and confirm for around 2 - a couple of of.5 hours or till the volume will increment in size concerning 1 half.
- Flip the batter onto a strip and cut, slide into the new preheated 450F/232.2C degree broiler onto a hot preparing stone, splash the mixture once with water rapidly, and afterward cover with a simmering top which has conjointly been preheated inside the stove. Prepare for 20 minutes.

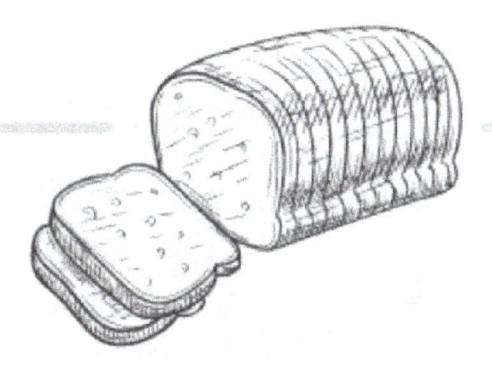

- After 20minutes, start the cooking top and turn down the broiler to 400F/204.4C degrees. Keep preparing for eighteen - 25 additional minutes or until your bread thermometer peruses 200 205F/93-96C. Flip the portion part of the way through the last heating sum for searing. Cool. For the ensuing portion, turn the stove back up to 450F/232.2C degrees and set the simmering top.

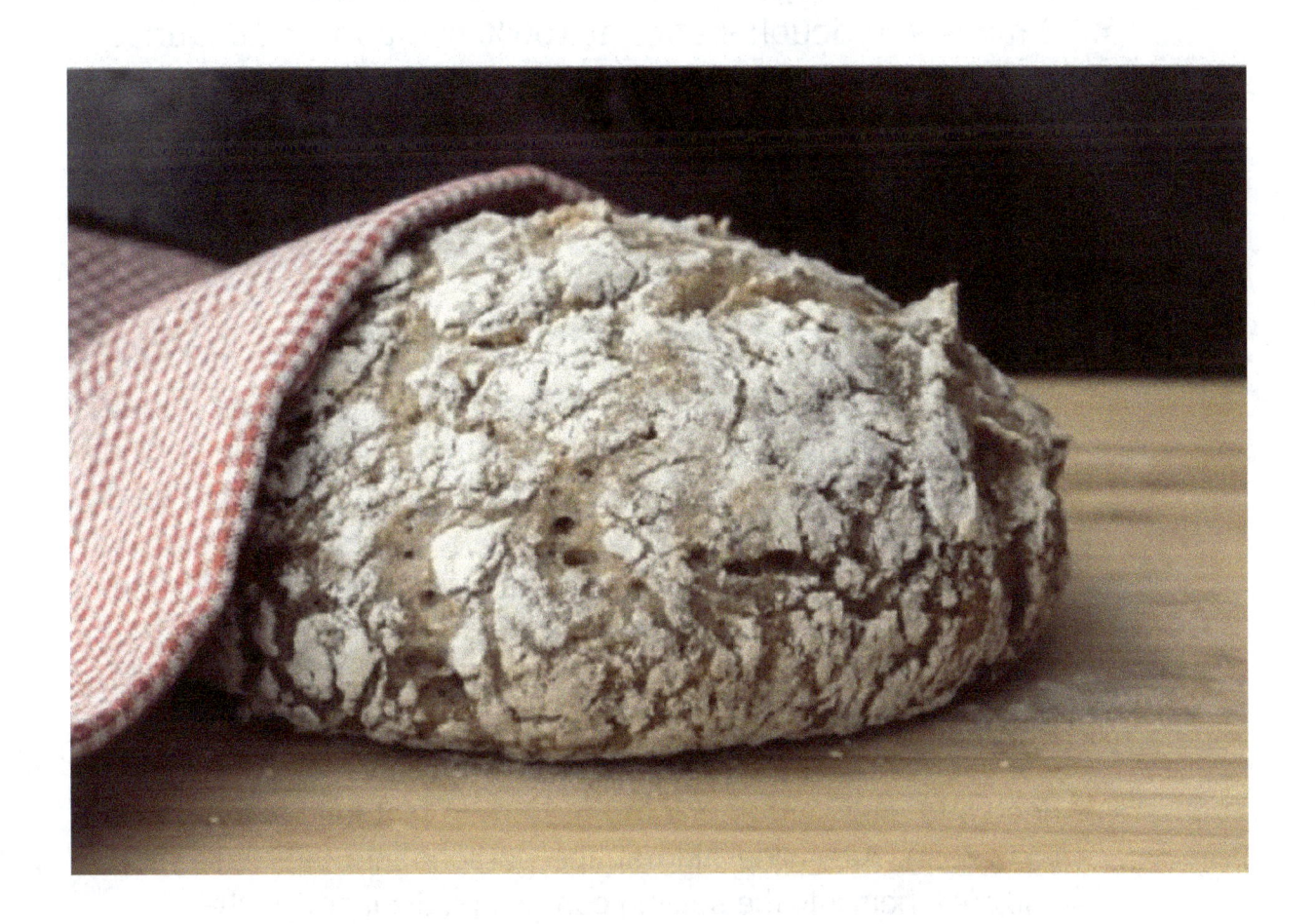

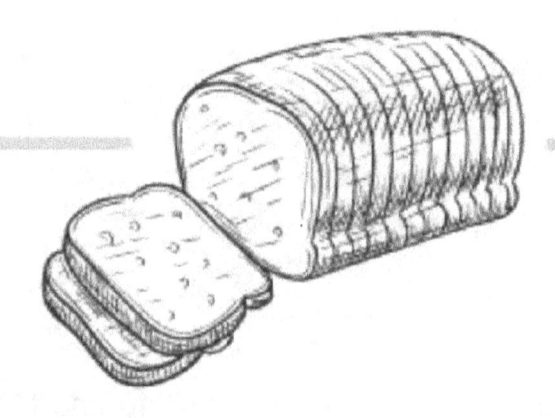

Westerham Farm Sourdough

Ingredients:

- 2 Tbsp butter melted and cooled – 1 Ounce
- 1 mug of Whole Wheat flour – 4.2 Ounce
- 6 one-fourth mugs Bread Flour – 28.1 Ounce
- 2 mugs sourdough starter at 166% hydration – 18 Ounce
- 1 one-fourth mugs water – 10 Ounce
- half mug of cream or half & half milk, scalded then cooled – 4 Ounce
- 4 tsp salt – .8 Ounce

Instructions:

- Consolidate all fixings, aside from salt, together until joined and afterward empower the mixture to rest for twenty minutes (batter autolysis). After mixture autolysis, add salt and join batter on low speed for around 2 minutes. At that point let the batter mass mature (introductory ascent) for six hours or until multiplied. Spot the mixture into a collapsing box and overlay it once every hour during massaging.
- After massaging, pour the batter onto a daintily floured surface and manipulate it enough to collect it into a ball. Gap the mixture into two things. Structure each portion into the overall shape you need and afterward permit the mixture to rest for 5 – ten minutes (seat rest). After sidelining shape portions into their last shapes and spot them into the sealing containers, dish, or Couche.
- Cover the mixture with plastic baggage and refrigerate for the time being. Toward the beginning of the day, permit the mixture

to definite confirmation for 2 – 3 hours (at whatever point the batter looks around one-half times its size and is elastic/springy) at that

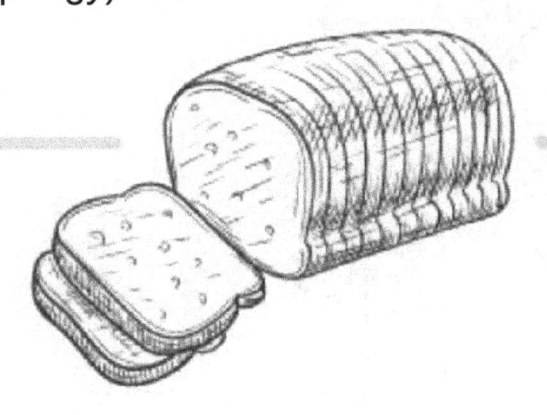

point turn mixture out on strip and slice, shower, cover with cooking top and heat in an extremely preheated 425F/218C degree broiler for twenty minutes.

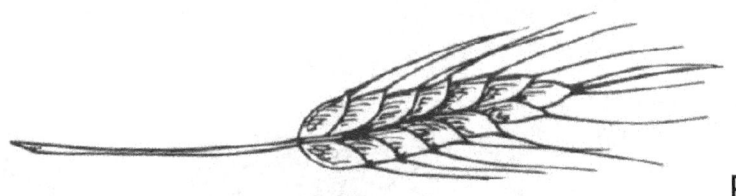

- Following twenty minutes, eliminate simmering top, flip down the broiler to 400F/204C degrees and keep heating for concerning ten-15 a lot of minutes, turning most of the way for cooking. Take out portion and cool on a rack. On the off chance that your first portion turns out excessively earthy colored, keep the temperature of the stove at 400F/204C degrees all through the full preparing period on the resulting heat. Remember to put the simmering cover once more into the broiler to preheat before setting up the ensuing portion.

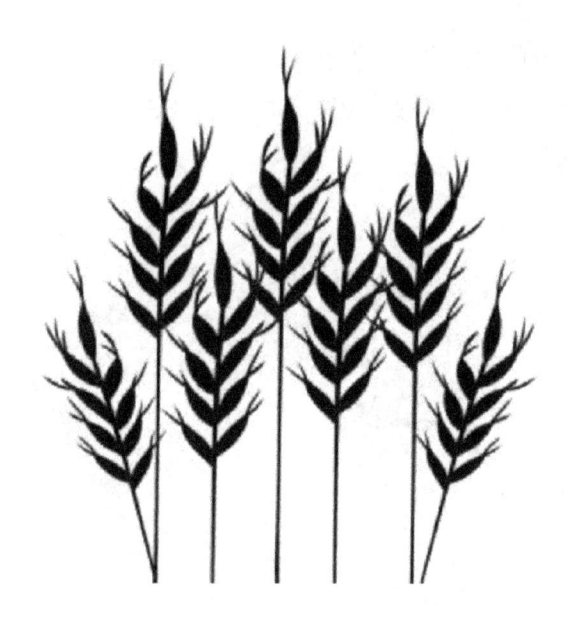

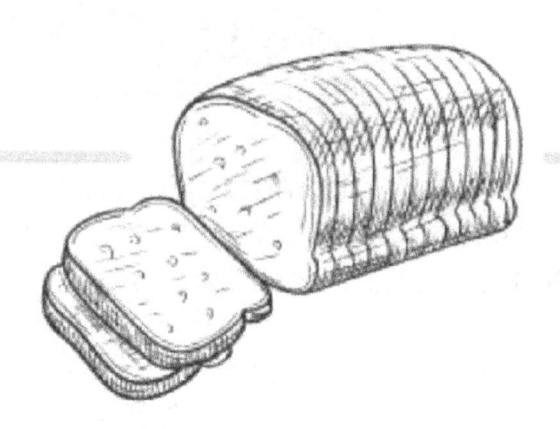

Ciabatta Sourdough
Ingredients:

- 1 Tablespoon Oil (.5 Ounce)
- 2.5 tsp salt added after dough autolysis (.5 Ounce)
- 18 Ounce 166% vigorous starter
- 6 Ounce water
- 3 Ounce canned milk
- 1 pound 6 Ounce of bread flour

Instructions:

- You'll have the option to make about a couple of portions at one pound of 9 Ounce each and along these lines, the completed mixture is at 70% hydration. Join along all fixings (except the salt), put for 3 minutes on low/medium speed in your Mixer. At that point let the batter sit for 20 minutes (autolysis).

- Add the salt and Combine the batter for five extra minutes, utilizing the base speed on your Mixer. Spot the batter during a collapsing box and let the mixture mature for four hours at zone temperature. When 60 minutes, mix or overlap the batter over on itself. After the batter is finished massaging, place it in the cooler short-term in an extremely lined holder. Next morning permit the mixture to warm up either at space temperature for two hours or in a sealing box (dishwasher) for one hour at around eighty-90F/26 32C degrees. At the point when the batter is heated up pour it onto an all-around floured surface. This mixture is kind of a thick player.

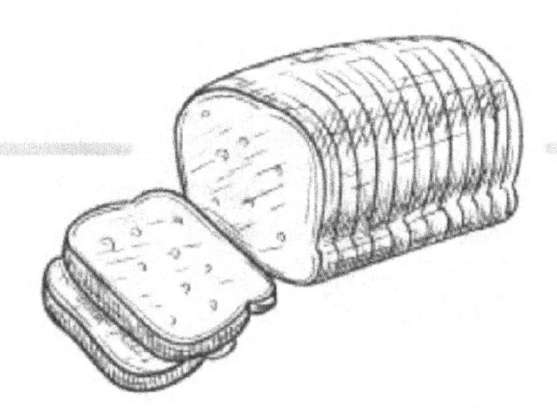

- Measure out concerning one pound of 8 Ounce of batter for each portion and spill this tacky protuberance out onto the intensely floured surface. The batter will resemble a thick mass on the prime of the flour. Presently crease the mixture over on prime of itself, keeping your hands just on the floured parts of the batter, it will harden up fairly. You don't have to work this batter since you wish to try not to add an exorbitant measure of flour to the wet mixture. Simply keep heaps of flour on the outside of the mixture to remain it from adhering to the table, if it sticks, strip it off alongside your baked good scrubber.

- Spot mixture onto a floured heating sheet or an intensely floured Couche. At the point when each portion is molded, let evidence for around 1 - 1.5 hours. When the portions are quite puffy, dimple the batter alongside your fingertips, squeezing them into the mixture to smooth it to some degree. Just before placing the batter into the broiler, take the portion and stretch it out a minuscule sum the long way, at that point prepare during a preheated stove at 450F/232C degrees for fifteen minutes, turn portions around and turn over right down to 425F/218C for an extra 15-18 minutes or till a profound brilliant earthy red. You can put your heating sheet straightforwardly onto the preparing stone, or you'll slide the portions off of the skillet and straightforwardly onto the stone (on the off chance that your container is level without any sides.

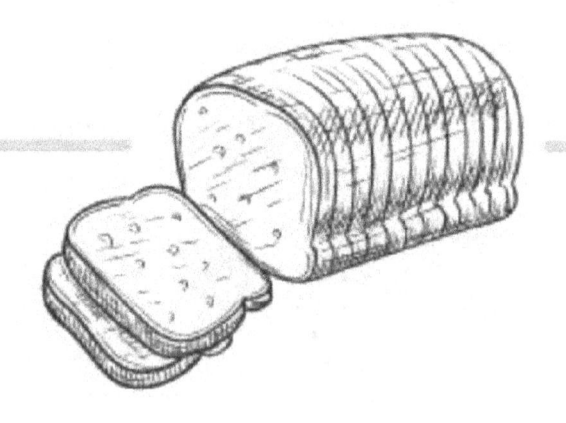

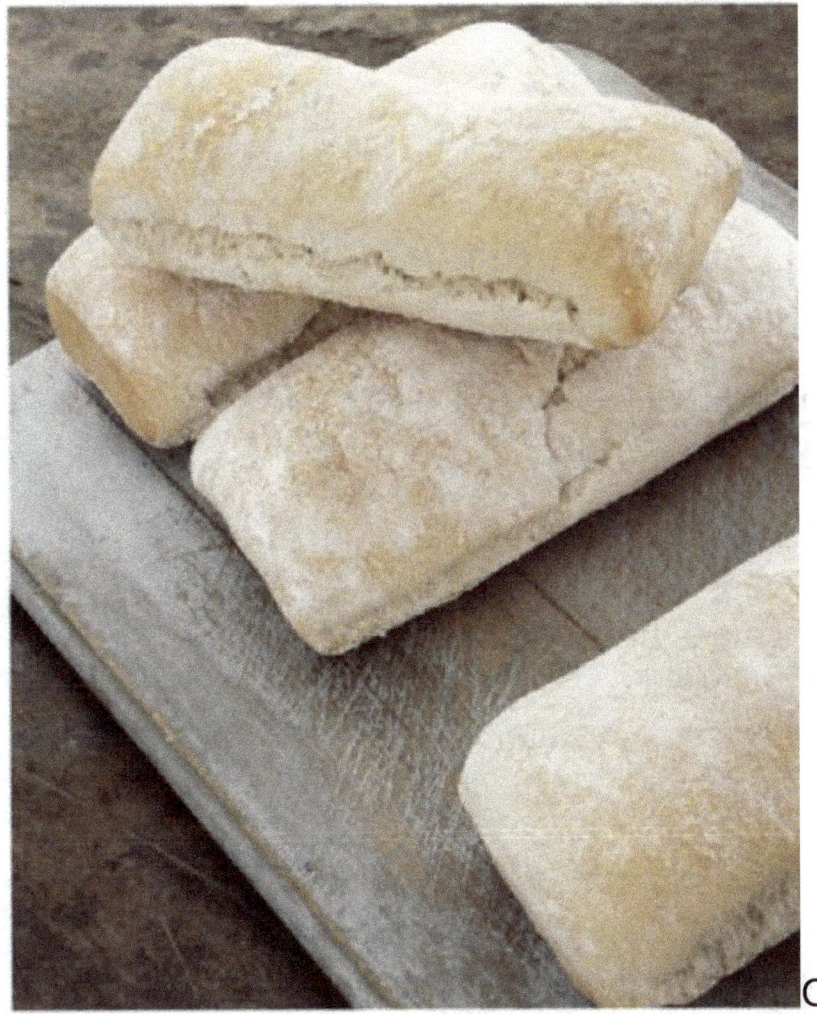

- On the off chance that you utilize a Couche, turn out your portions onto an all-around floured strip and spot into the new broiler straightforwardly onto the hot stone. If you'll have the option to cover the mixture with a simmering top for the essential 12 minutes, that may work considerably higher, in any case, don't splash the portions with water, simply permit the steam from the batter to attempt to do the undertaking.

Cool portions and afterward cut and present with loads of margarine.

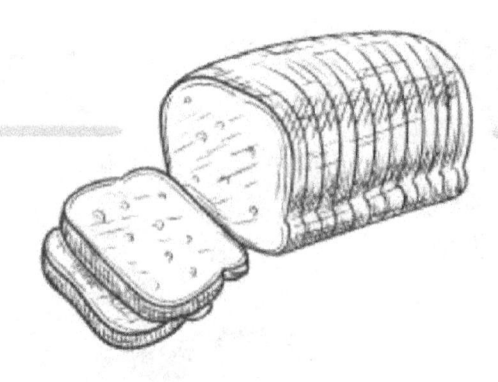

Hearth Flaxseed Sourdough

Ingredients:

- 2/3 mug rye Flour- 2.4 Ounce
- 3 mugs whole wheat flour – 12.6
- 1/3 mugs bread flour 1 Pound 3.4 Ounce
- 2 mugs active sourdough starter – 18 Ounce
- 2 mugs warm water – 16 Ounce
- 2 TBSP Oil – 1 Ounce
- 2 TBSP malt syrup – 1.6 Ounce
- 1/4 mug cornmeal – 1.2 Ounce
- 4 tsp salt (add salt after dough autolysis) - .8 Ounce

Instructions:

- Interaction fixings in your Mixer on speed two or medium speed, for concerning two minutes, till fixings are consolidated. At that point Dough autolysis for twenty minutes. After Dough autolysis adds salt and Combine for an additional two minutes. Then, massage for six hours at space temperature. While mass maturing, you'll either utilize a batter collapsing box (see Dough Folding) or keep the mixture in your Mixer and overlap the mixture once consistently. On the off chance that you keep your mixture in your Mixer, flip your Mixer on low and turn down the batter once an hour utilizing just 3 turns of the snare.
- Consolidate the seeds and wheat into the batter well, either by hand or at low-speed on the off chance that you kept your mixture inside the Mixer. Spot mixture on rye floured surface, manipulate now and then (barely to assemble into a ball), partition batter into two things.

•

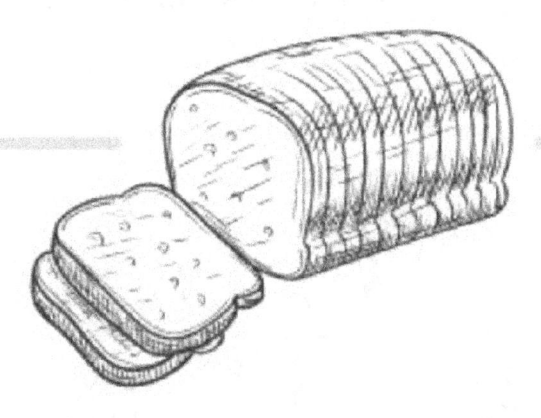

Shape the batter into the last shape you want it to be and allow it to rest for five – 10 minutes. At that point do a last forming of the portions and spot them into sealing bannetons or containers fixed with a sealing material and sprinkled with rye flour. Cowl the entire container with a plastic sack. Refrigerate for the time being. Inside the morning eliminates your portions forty minutes separated and let them warm up till sealed and arranged to prepare (one. Five - three hours).

- On the off chance that you need to put Flax seeds on the high of the outside layer: beat one egg with one Tablespoon of water, brush this egg Mixture over the portions and sprinkle with Flax seeds. Cut mixture. Spot mixture during a preheated 425F/218C degree stove, onto a hot heating stone. Working rapidly… Spray the mixture all over once with water, and afterward cowl the batter with a broiling cover which has conjointly been preheated in the broiler. Prepare for twenty minutes, at that point get going the cooking cover and turn down the stove to 400F/204C degrees.
- Keep preparing for twenty - 25 additional minutes, turning the portion once for cooking. The bread should enroll 200 205F/93-96C degrees on a prompt thermometer. For the following portion, turn the stove back up to 425F/218C degrees and spot the simmering cover back in to preheat until the portion is set up to go in. Heat equivalent to the essential portion.

Cool and appreciate slathered with a new spread. This bread makes stupendous toast and sandwiches.

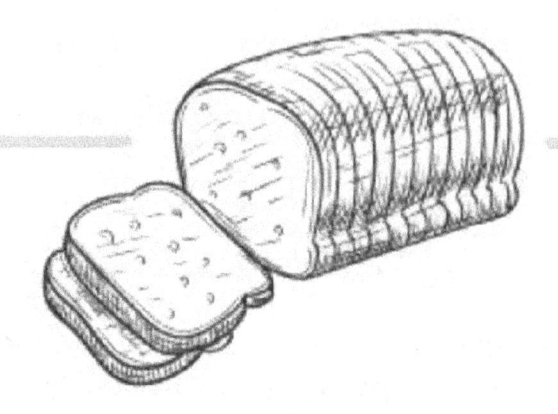

Light Onion Rye Sourdough

Ingredients:

- 3 Tbsp dried onion flakes – .6
- 2 Tbsp Caraway seeds – 0.5 Ounce
- 1 half tsp granulated onion – .1
- 3 half tsp salt – .7 Ounce
- 2 mugs Rye flour – 7.2 Ounce
- 2 mugs vigorous sourdough starter
- 1third-fourth mugs water – 14 Ounce
- 2 Tbsp Oil – 1.0 Ounce
- 1 Tablespoon Malt syrup – 0.8 Ounce
- 2 mugs Whole Wheat flour –8.4 Ounce
- 3 mugs Bread flour (approximately) – 13.5 Ounce

Instructions:

- Combine all ingredients except salt for two-three minutes till well combined. Dough autolysis and then add salt.
- Combine for one more minute to combine within the salt. Let proof for four - half-drunken hours or until doubled. Pour dough out on a gently floured (Whole Wheat or Rye flour works best) surface and knead into a ball about four to 5 kneads. Separate into two items and form every part into a loaf. Place loaves the wrong way up in bowls or baskets lined with a proofing cloth

and sprinkled with Rye flour.
- Cover with a plastic bag and place within the refrigerator overnight. In the morning eliminate each loaf 40 minutes apart, uncover and let rise (a pair of - three hours or until prepared).

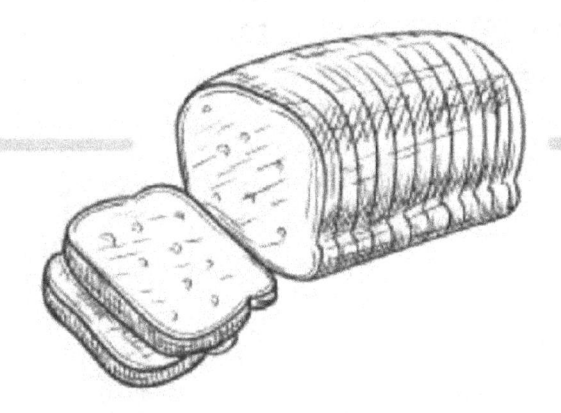

Wholegrain Sourdough

Ingredients:

- 1 mug Rye flour – 3.6 Ounce/102 g
- 1 teaspoon salt - .2 Ounce/5.7
- 3 mugs sifted Spring Wheat flour
- 1 mug whole wheat starter
- 2 mugs water – 16 Ounce/453 g

Instructions:

- Spill out the mixture onto a delicately floured (Rye or Wheat flour) surface and massage various occasions, at that point assemble into a ball. Allow mixture to rest for ten minutes and afterward do the last forming. Spot the mixture into the sealing crate, which is fixed with a sealing material (Bannetons don't should be lined). Put the container of the mixture, coconut trainer pack, inside containers-term.
- Next morning dispose of portion and grant to evidence one – three hours or until arranged to heat. At the point when the batter is arranged and feels effervescent and springy anyway not droopy, at that point take the portion and sprinkle the top (actually the base) with semolina or entire grain flour and turn the mixture out onto a strip of level heating sheet. At that point

slice the mixture while still on the strip, slide into the hot preheated 450F/232C degree stove onto a hot heating stone, splash the batter once with water rapidly, and afterward cover with a simmering top that has additionally been preheated inside the broiler. Heat for 20 minutes. Following 20 minutes, start the simmering cover and flip down the broiler to 400F/204C degrees.

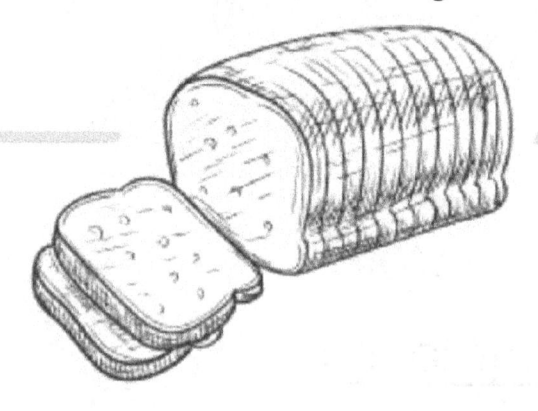

- Keep heating for concerning forty additional minutes, turning the portion once for searing. To construct certain the portion is done, utilizing your bread thermometer, look at to work if it's at 200-205F/93-96C degrees inside the focal point of the portion.
- If the outside layer appears to get excessively earthy colored through heating, cover the top gently with a piece of foil. Micha is ideal whenever left to chill off totally and it improves in flavor and surface since it will so. Eat with masses of ongoing spread and additionally cream cheddar.

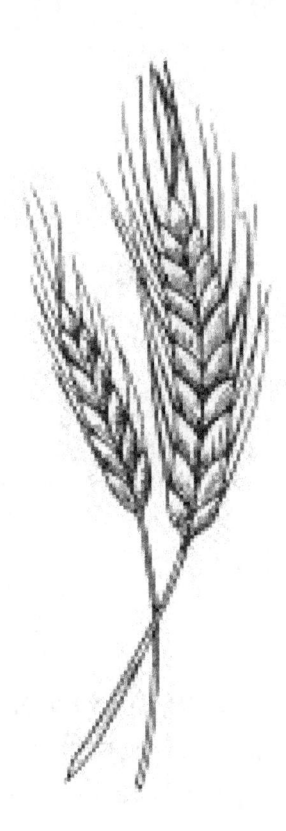

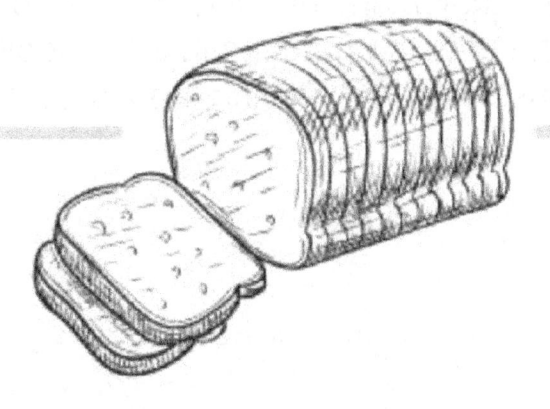

Ripped Pumpkin Sourdough

Ingredients:

- Tablespoon Oil – 1 Ounce
- 1 heaping Tablespoon malt syrup or honey – 1 Ounce
- 4 half mugs Bread flour – 20.2 Ounce bread flour- you can use part all-purpose flour
- 1 mug ripe, vigorous starter
- 1 half mugs water – 12 Ounce
- 3 mugs bread flour – 13.5 Ounce
- 3 half tsp salt (add after dough autolysis) - .7 Ounce

Instructions:

- Consolidate the entirety of the fixings until joined. Utilize the low or medium speed setting on your Mixer. When the fixings have been joined together, turn off your Mixer and permit the mixture autolysis (rest) for 20 minutes. After the batter autolysis period, flip your Mixer back on the most reduced speed and add the .9 Ounce of salt. Allow the mixture to consolidate at low speed for around four minutes to build up the gluten.
- The mixture will be tacky. Spot the mixture back into a batter collapsing box on the off chance that you have one or a goliath compartment and let it mature for four hours until around eleven:30 am. In the case of utilizing the collapsing box, overlap the batter about once an hour to fortify the gluten.
- When maturing for four hours, take the batter and gap it into 2 things. At that point utilizing an all-around floured surface shape and spot the portions into the sealing containers, fixed with intensely floured sealing fabrics, or utilize a Couche.

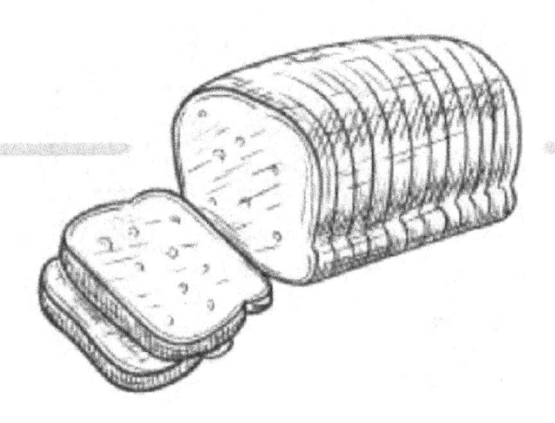

To amaze the portions, shape the second portion thirty minutes after the essential portion, subsequently, they will be heated on various occasions. Permit portions to conclusive evidence, that should take one – 2 hours. When there is about an hour until heating time, preheat your broiler to 450F/232.2C degrees. At the point when the mixture is arranged and feels effervescent and springy, take the primary portion and turn the batter out onto a strip of level preparing sheet. Press pumpkin seeds into the prime of the batter and slice if you wish.

- Slide into the hot preheated 450F/232.2C degree broiler, onto a hot heating stone, splash the mixture once with water rapidly, and afterward cover with a simmering top that has moreover been preheated in the stove. Prepare for twenty minutes. Following twenty minutes, start the simmering top and flip down the broiler to 400F/204.4C degrees. Keep heating for 15 - 20 extra minutes, turning the portion once for sautéing. To fabricate positive the portion is done, utilizing your bread thermometer, check to decide whether it's at 200-205F/93-96C degrees in the focal point of the portion.
- For the following portion, turn the stove duplicate 450F/232.2C degrees, and set the simmering cover back into preheat. Heat equivalent to the essential portion. This bread could be a light pumpkin-shaded, the ethereal portion with crunchy cooked seeds on the high outside layer. It will fabricate an extraordinary Halloween buffet portion.

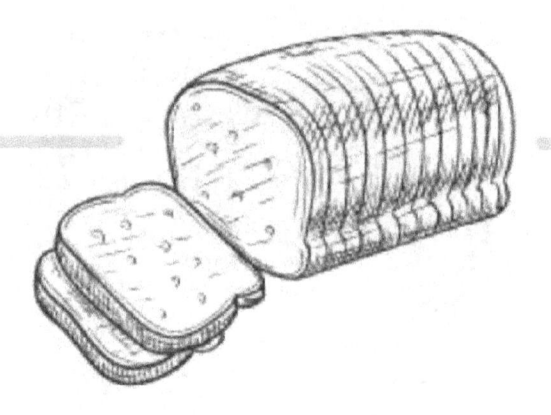

Rich Egg and Butter Sourdough

Ingredients:

- 1⁄2 mug room temperature
- water
- 1⁄4 mug heavy cream
- 2 eggs
- 1 tablespoon sugar
- 3 mugs (131⁄2 ounces) sourdough
- flour, plus more as needed
- 21⁄4 tsp active dry yeast
- 1 teaspoon kosher salt
- 8 tbsp unsalted butter,
- at room temperature
- Nonstock baking spray
- Egg wash (1 egg Combined with
- 1 tablespoon water; optional)

Instructions:

- Consolidate the flour, yeast, water, genuine cream, eggs, and sugar during a stand Mixer fitted with the mixture snare and ply until the batter is wash.
- Add the salt and spread, each tablespoon in turn, manipulating until the margarine is consolidated without fail. Cover the bowl with cling wrap and let the mixture ascend till it's multiplied in size, for one hour in a warm room. In the interim, shower a 9 x 5-inch portion skillet with a heating splash.

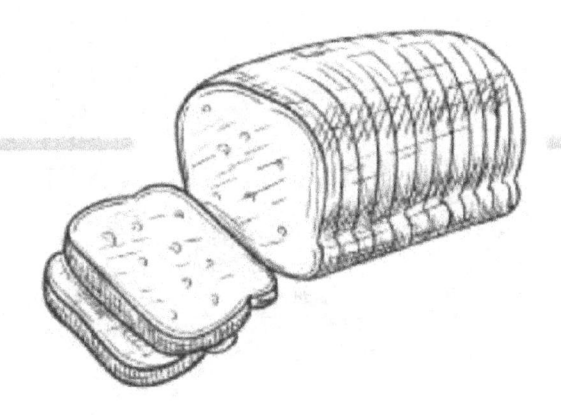

Turn the batter out onto a tenderly floured surface and pat it into a harsh 8-inch sq. Overlap the prime in regard to the focal point of the mixture and press the edge directly down to get it.

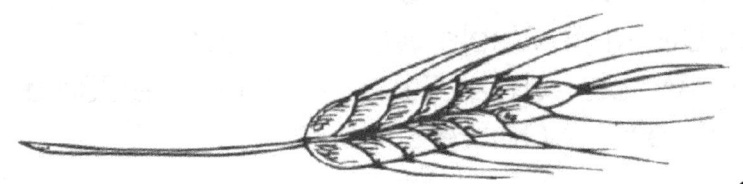

- Crease the high over again, this chance to inside concerning an inch or along these lines of the base. Press the edge to seal. Presently pull the lower part of the batter up to fulfill the mixture roll you've made and seal the crease. Squeeze the closures shut and place the batter, crease aspect down, in the prepared portion dish.
- Cover the skillet with saran wrap or spot the full dish in a goliath plastic sack and tie the open completion shut. Refrigerate for the time being or up to 24 hours before heating. The mixture ought to completely rise once concerning 6 hours; nonetheless, a more drawn-out rest is sweet for it.

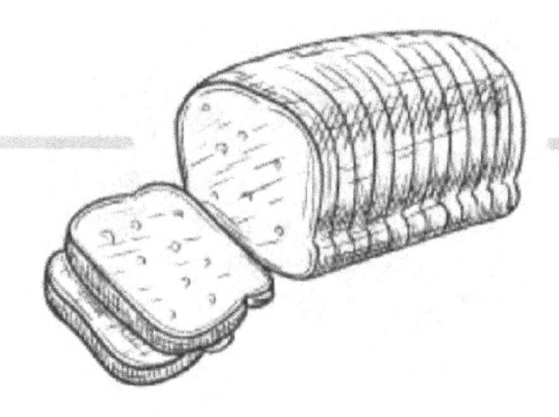

Spelt Walter Sourdough

Ingredients:

- 3 half mugs Whole Spelt Flour – 12 .2 Ounce/345.9 g
- 2 half mugs water – 20 Ounce/567 g
- 1 mug Deem or Whole Wheat starter
- 2 mugs Whole Wheat Flour – 8.4 Ounce/238 g
- 1 tsp of salt - .2 Ounce/5.7 g

Instructions:

- Consolidate the fixings on a medium speed essentially until joined, this takes in regards to two minutes. At that point grant the mixture autolysis (rest) for twenty minutes. After autolysis, consolidate batter on low speed for concerning 4 minutes. At that point let the mixture massage (which just recommends that the essential ascent) for 3 – four hours till multiplied. After massaging, spill out the batter onto a gently floured (Spelt flour) surface and two or multiple times, at that point assemble into a ball.
- Gap the mixture into 2 or 3 pieces. Amaze the forming of the portions thirty minutes separated. Shape portions into the last shape you wish and afterward license the batter to rest for 10 minutes (seat rest). After resting, structure portions into their last shapes and spot them into the sealing bushels, or skillet that is fixed with sealing fabrics on the off chance that you wish (Bannetons don't ought to be lined). License the mixture to ascend till sealing is done. Sealing is that the second raising of the mixture. For this formula, it can take around 1.5 – 2 hours. At

the point when the mixture is arranged and feels effervescent and springy anyway not droopy, at that point taking the principal portion sprinkle the high (genuinely the underside) with

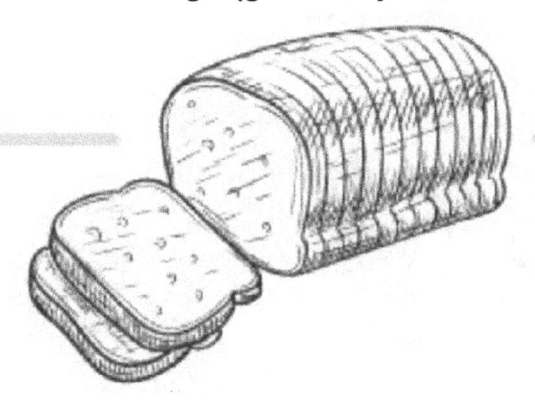

semolina or entire grain flour and flip the batter out onto a strip of level preparing sheet. At that point cut the batter while still on the strip, slide into the hot preheated 450F/232C degree stove onto a hot preparing stone, splash the mixture once with water rapidly, and afterward cover with a cooking top which has also been preheated inside the broiler. Heat for twenty minutes.

Following 20 minutes, get going the cooking top and turn down the broiler to 425F/218C degrees. Keep preparing for 15-20 additional minutes, turning the portion once for sautéing. For the resulting portion, flip the stove back up and place the simmering top back in to preheat for five minutes until the portion is prepared to go in. Prepare equivalent to the primary portion. Cool this flavorful bread and eat with late margarine. Sourdough Spelt Bread incorporates a chewy hull and a delicate, soggy scrap and is incredible for sandwiches or toast or to eat new with cream cheddar.

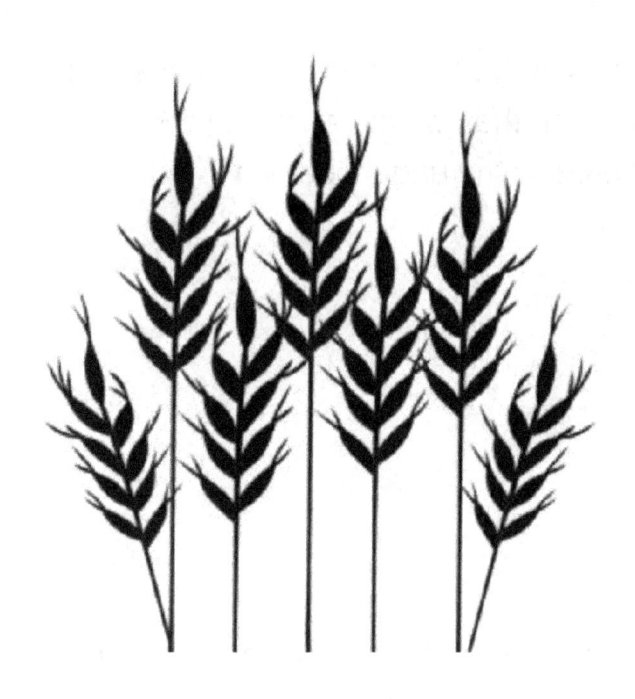

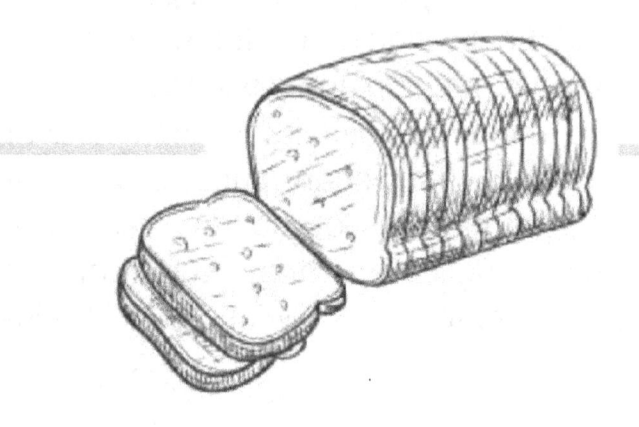

Extra Sour Sourdough
Ingredients:

- half mug Rye Flour – 1.8 – Ounce
- half mug Whole Wheat flour – 2.1 Ounce
- 6 one-fourth mugs Bread flour –1 pound. 12 Ounce

- 2 mugs vigorous sourdough starter 1third-
- fourth mugs water tepid water– 14.0 Ounce 1
- Tablespoon oil – .5 Ounce
- 1 teaspoon diastatic malt powder - .1Ounce
- 3.5 tsp salt - .7 Ounce (add after autolyze)

Instructions:

- Join the fixings well in your Combiner for concerning two - 3 minutes or just until Combined. At that point permit the mixture to autolyze (rest) for twenty minutes. After autolysis, add salt and Combine the mixture at a low speed for around 1 moment. At that point let the mixture massage (which simply recommends that the essential ascent) for six -eight hours in a warm 80F/twenty-six.7C spot.
- Mix the batter down with only 3 turns of the mixture snare multiple times all through the 6 - 8-hour massaging or crease the batter in a collapsing box. This is to fortify the gluten strands and line them up in addition to it assists with remaining the batter from over aging. After mass maturation, pour the mixture onto a delicately floured surface and two or multiple times at that point assemble into a ball. Separation the mixture into two pieces.

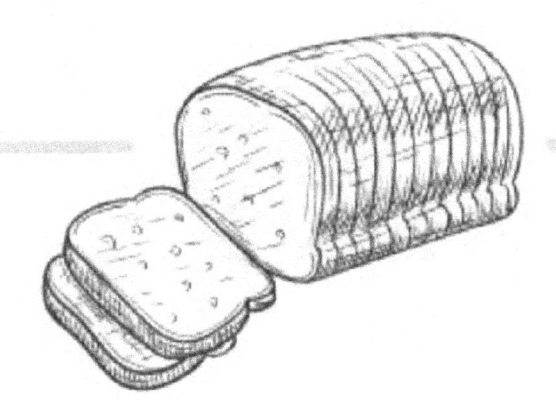

- Structure portions into the general structure you need and afterward grant the batter to rest for five - 10 minutes (seat rest). After sidelining shape portions into their last shapes and put them into the sealing bushels, or containers which are fixed with sealing fabrics (Bannetons don't should be lined). Permit the batter to set out for a half-hour and afterward refrigerate, covered

with plastic stuff, short-term.
- You can avoid the half-hour pause if the mixture has been vivacious during the day. The next morning eliminate the portions thirty minutes separated (so you don't need to heat them simultaneously) at that point empower the batter to ascend until it is finished sealing. This can take somewhere in the range of one-three hours and is the point at which the mixture increments in size around one-half times. At the point when the mixture is prepared and feels effervescent and springy anyway not droopy, at that point taking the essential portion sprinkle the top (actually the underside) with semolina or entire grain flour and flip out onto a strip of level heating sheet.
- At that point slice the mixture while it is as yet on the strip, slide the batter into the new preheated 450F/232.2C degree stove onto a hot heating stone, shower the batter once with water rapidly, and afterward cowl with a cooking cover which has moreover been preheated in the broiler. Heat for 20 minutes.

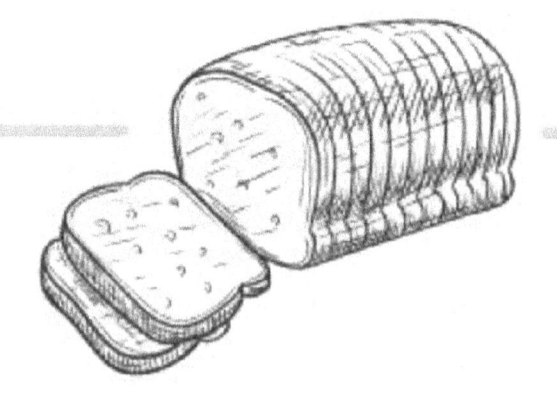

Berlin Style Sharp
Ingredients:

- one-fourth mug whole wheat flour- 1
- Ounce 1 mug ripe, vigorous starter 1
- half mugs water – 12 Ounce

- 3 mugs bread flour – 13.5

Ounce **Instructions:**

- Consolidate all fixings together mixture autolysis with salt until all-around joined, this can take concerning two - 3 minutes. Empower the mixture to rest for 20 minutes. At the point when the rest of, flip your Mixer back on the least speed consolidate for an additional two minutes. The mixture can be tacky. Spot the mixture back into a collapsing compartment and let it age until 9:00 pm, collapsing batter once consistently. At that point place the holder into the cooler short-term.
- Keep something contrary to the mixture shrouded with plastic or in a covered compartment to hold it back from drying out. At that point, thirty minutes after the fact shape the subsequent portion. Empower the two portions to warm up and do their last confirmation, this should take two-three hours, or until the portion looks one-half times its unique size. Preheat your broiler to 450F/232.2C degrees when there is about an hour left until heating time.
- At the point when the mixture is arranged and feels effervescent and springy, take the essential portion sprinkle the prime (really, the underside) with semolina, and flip the batter out onto a strip of level preparing sheet.

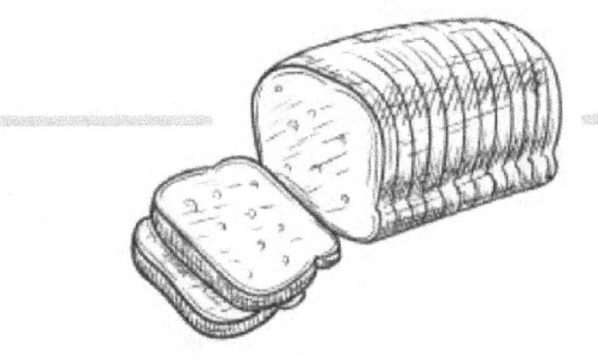

At that point cut the batter while still on the strip, slide into the hot preheated 450F/232.2C degree stove onto a hot preparing stone, splash the mixture once with water rapidly, and afterward cover with a broiling top which has furthermore been preheated inside the broiler. Prepare for twenty minutes. When 20minutes, kick off the cooking cover and turn down the broiler to 425F/218C degrees. Keep heating for 15 additional minutes, turning the portion once for searing. To construct positive the portion is done, utilizing your bread thermometer, look at to work if it's at 200 205F/93 96C degrees inside the focal point of the portion.

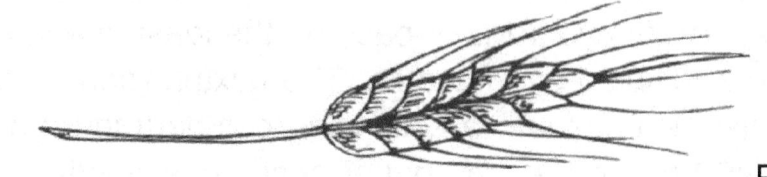

- For the accompanying portion, turn the broiler copy to 450F/232.2C degrees and set the cooking cover back into preheat. Prepare the indistinguishable as the primary portion. This bread is best after being cooled for a few hours to permit the harshness to create. The severe tang will grow even up till the next day.

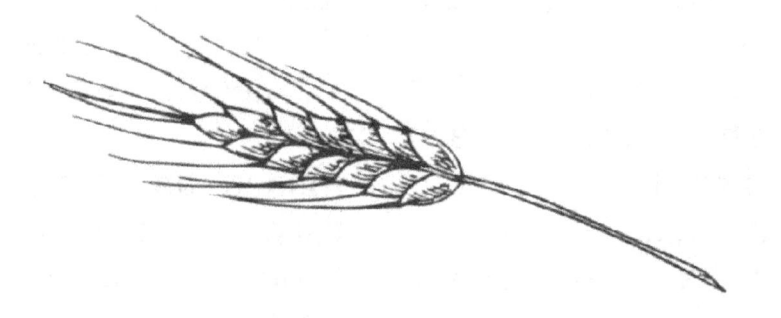

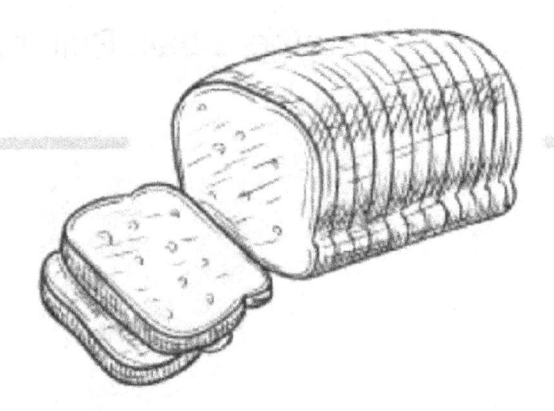

Sour Malt Sourdough

Ingredients:

- 1 pound 13.3 Ounce of bread flour
- 2 heaping Tbsp Malt syrup- add after dough autolysis
- 1 mug sourdough starter
- 2 half mugs water – 20 Ounce
- 3 tsp salt- add after dough autolysis- .6 Ounce

Instructions:

- Retain 6 Ounces of the water, the malt syrup, and subsequently the salt. This is accordingly you'll have the option to utilize the Double Hydration Method that you'll examine inside the Advanced segment. Consolidate along with all fixings (aside from 6Ounce of water, malt syrup, and hence the salt) for concerning 3 minutes on low/medium speed in your Mixer. At that point let the batter sit for twenty minutes (mixture autolysis). Presently add the salt and join the batter for 4 extra minutes, utilizing the base speed on your Mixer. Around the finish of the four minutes of joining, gradually add the 6 Ounces of water and the malt syrup and Combine a brief more.
- Spot the batter in an incredibly monster-covered holder and let the mixture mature for the time being at zone temperature. Next morning, gauge the mixture into two pieces, you will require a bowl or plate for weighing wet, tacky batter. Each piece ought to weigh roughly 1pound 14 Ounce or subsequently. The batter is tacky with dashes of malt syrup in it. Take the gauged batter and keeping it inside the gauging bowl or plate, start pulling up the

edges and sides to frame a ball. Pull from the surface and squeeze to within the ball.

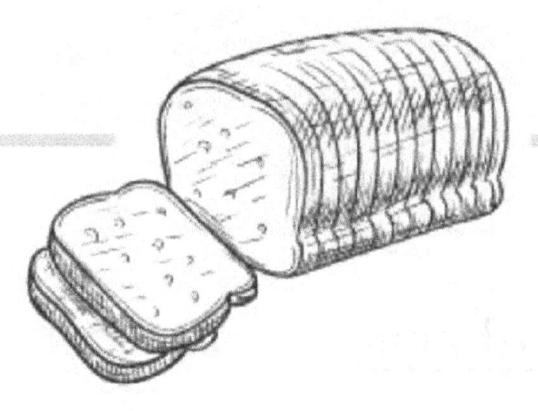

- The mixture is incredibly wet and difficult to deal with. At the point when it is fairly framed into a ball, thud the wet bundle of the mixture into the focal point of the texture-lined container, assemble certain the sealing material is very much floured with semolina flour. Rapidly cowl the remainder of the batter ball with a weighty sprinkling of semolina flour, before it's an opportunity to unfurl and come in contact with the texture on the borders. Confirmation mixture for 2 hours at zone temperature. At the point when the batter has been sealing for 60 minutes, turn on your over to preheat to 450F/232C degrees and remember to preheat your simmering lies.

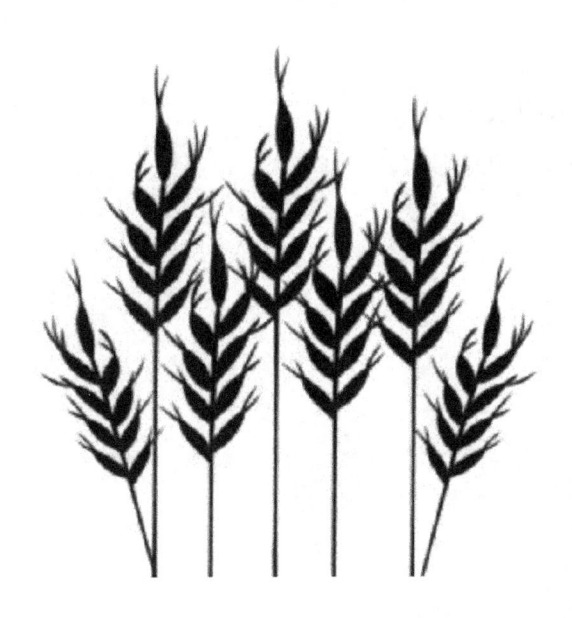

Kalamata Asiago Sourdough
Ingredients:

- 5 mugs Bread flour –1 pound 6.5 Ounce/637.9 g
- 3 tsp salt – .6 Ounce/17 g
- Use these ingredients when rolling up the dough:
- Kalamata Olives –12 Ounce/340 g
- Asiago Cheese – 8 Ounce/226 g
- White sourdough starter
- Rye Starter at 100% hydration – 5 Ounce/141 g
- half mug water – 4 Ounce/113 g

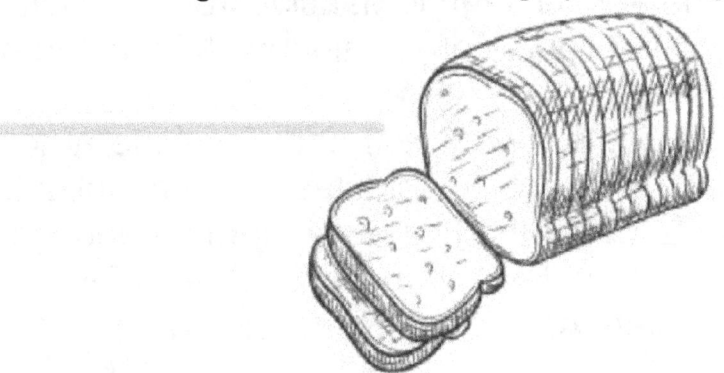

- half mug evaporated Milk – 4
- Ounce/113 g 2 Tbsp oil – 1 Ounce/28 g
- Fresh Rosemary chopped – 1 Ounce/28 g

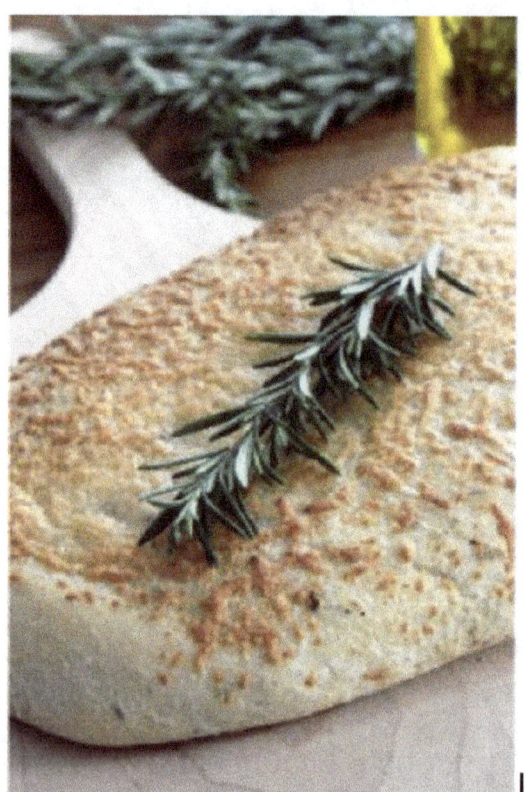

Instructions:

- In the principal morning, utilizing your mixture Mixer, Combine the entirety of the fixings inside the excellent rundown aside from the salt. This should take about a couple of - 3 minutes. Mixture autolysis for 20 minutes.
- At that point add your salt and Combine at low speed for around five a lot of minutes the consolidating for this mixture is longer than for a standard sourdough, since it's a 1-day batter and will not go through as a few hours building up the gluten. After it is finished joining,

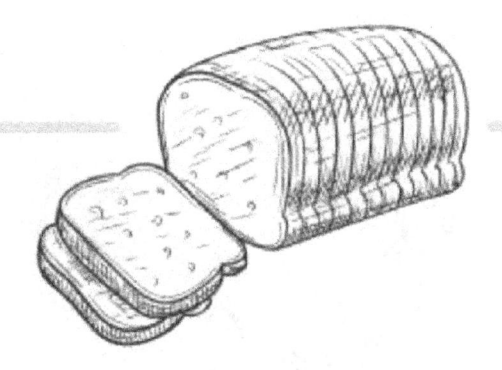

flip the batter out into a mixture collapsing box or holder.

- Permit this batter to mass mature six hours and overlap it about once 60 minutes. You'll really, see the mixture get more grounded with each collapsing. After six hours of mass maturation, partition the batter into two things weighing around one-pound 11Ounce/765 g each. Let the mixture things set for 5-ten minutes. Planned forming of the portions 30 minutes separated, accordingly that they will not be sealed simultaneously. Next get out the cheddar, olives, and new Rosemary. Channel the olives, 3D squares the cheddar, and slash the Rosemary leaves.

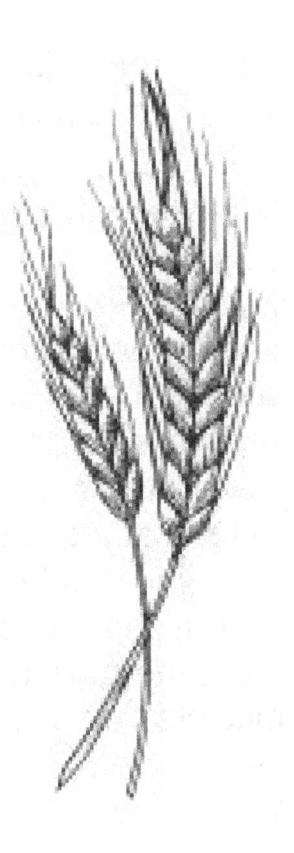

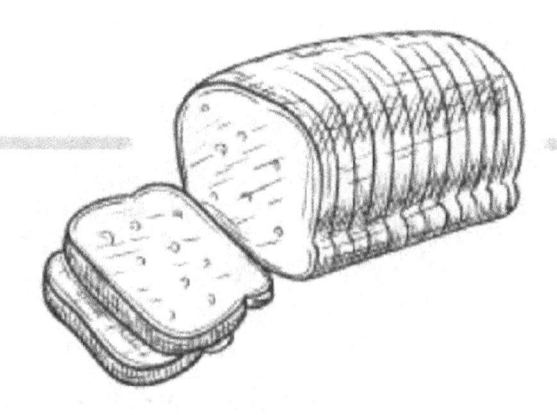

Cracked Wheat Borough Sourdough
Ingredients:

- 1/3 mug cracked wheat – 1.8 Ounce 6third-
- fourth mugs bread flour –1 pound 14.3 Ounce 4
- tsp salt – .8 Ounce
- 2 mugs sourdough starter 1third-fourth
- mugs tepid water – 14 Ounce 2 Tbsp
- oil - 1 Ounce

Instructions:

- Consolidate the fixings, except salt, on a medium speed just until joined, this takes concerning a few minutes. At that point license the mixture autolysis (rest) for twenty minutes.
- After autolysis, add salt and afterward consolidate the mixture on low speed for concerning 1 extra moment. At that point let the mixture mass mature (which simply implies the main ascent) for 7-8 hours or until multiplied. Overlay the batter multiple times during the massage which creates and lines up the gluten strands. If you are maturing your mixture inside the Mixer, hit the beginning catch and let the snare mix the batter about twice around the bowl on an untouched low setting. Or on the other hand, if utilizing a batter collapsing holder, overlay the mixture about each one-half hour or along these lines and cover. After mass maturation, spill out the mixture onto a tenderly floured surface and two or multiple times, at that point accumulate into a ball.

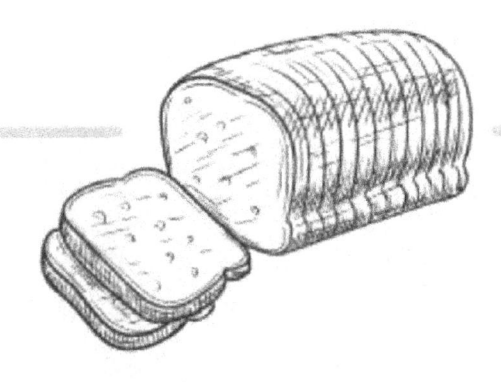

- Separation the batter into two things weighing around 2 pounds each. Shape portions into the general structure you need and afterward license the batter to rest for ten minutes (seat rest). After sidelining, shape portions into their last shapes and put them into the sealing crates, or container which is fixed with sealing fabrics (Bannetons don't should be lined). Let mixture dispatched for concerning 30 minutes and afterward cowl the batter with plastic baggage and refrigerate for the time being. Toward the beginning of the day, permit the batter to definite evidence for 2 - 3 hours (at whatever point the mixture looks around one-half times the main size) at that point turn the batter out on a strip. Slice, shower, cowl with simmering top and prepare in an extremely preheated 450F/232C degree stove for 20 minutes. Following 20 minutes, eliminate the cooking cover, turn the broiler directly down to 425F/218C degrees and keep heating for around fifteen additional minutes or until your bread thermometer peruses 200 205F/93-96C, turning most of the way for caramelizing.
- Take out a portion and cool on a rack. If your first portion turns out excessively earthy colored, turn the broiler directly down to 400F/204C degrees during the second of the heat rather than 425F/218C degrees. Remember to place the cooking cover into the stove and warm to 450F/232C degrees again, before fitting the following portion. This San Francisco Sourdough portion is chewy, consolidates a firm outside layer, and is loaded up with openings, it tastes decent!

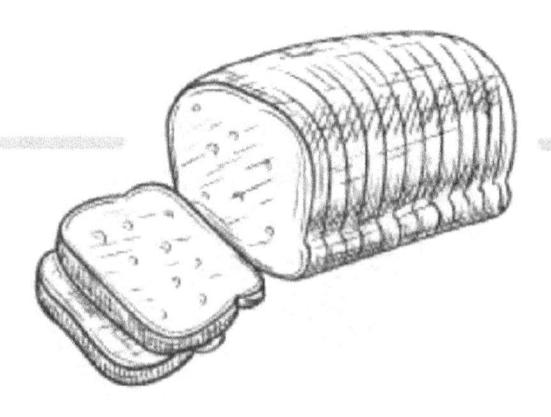

Northwestern Sourdough

Ingredients:

- half mug evaporated canned milk – 4.0 Ounce
- 1 Tablespoon Malt syrup - .8 Ounce
- 7&2/3 mugs Bread flour – 34 Ounce
- half mug vigorous sourdough starter – 4.5 Ounce
- 1 mug 166% hydration Northwest starter – 9.0 Ounce
- 1 & half mugs water– 12.0 Ounce
- 4 tsp salt – .8 Ounce (add after dough autolysis)

Instructions:

- Consolidate the entirety of the fixings (aside from the salt) well in your Mixer concerning 2 – 3 minutes on low speed or simply till joined. At that point empower the mixture autolysis (rest) for 20 minutes. After autolysis, add salt and afterward consolidate mixture at low speed for five minutes. Bread made with a 1 day consolidate and heat recipe should be joined longer to build up the gluten. Empower the mixture to mass mature (that implies that the essential ascent) for 4 hours.
- Mix the mixture down with only three turns of the batter snare twice all through the four-hour mass maturation. This is to reinforce the gluten strands and line them up, plentiful like collapsing would do. After massaging, pour the batter onto a daintily floured (Whole Wheat flour) surface and massage various occasions at that point assemble into a ball. Gap the batter into four pieces.

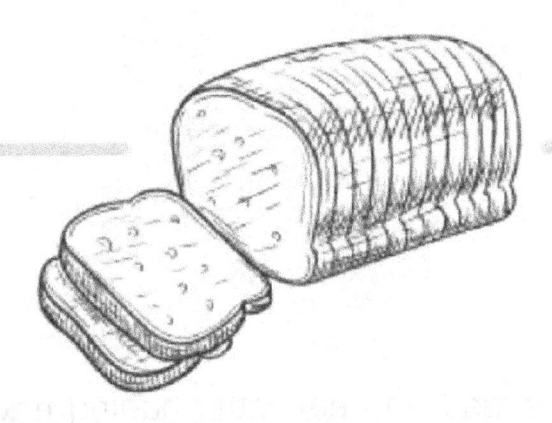

- Structure the mixture into thick ropes that are around 18 inches in length and afterward permit the batter to rest for five – 10 minutes (seat rest). In the wake of resting, structure portions into their last shapes by taking two things of the rope molded batter and bending them around each other. Wrap the winds up under the batter. Spot the portions into the sealing containers, or dish which are fixed with floured sealing fabrics. Stun the preparation of the portions by putting one portion inside the cooler for forty minutes. Verification of the batter for 1.5 – 2 hours during a warm place at 80F/26C. Either keep the sealing box damp or cowl the portions with soggy fabrics or plastic gear to hold the mixture back from drying out. Preheat your stove, preparing stone and broiling cover to 425F/218C degrees when you have concerning an hour left for sealing.
- At the point when the mixture is arranged and feels effervescent and springy yet not droopy, at that point taking the essential portion, tenderly do it of the banneton and spot it on a floured strip. Slice the mixture along with the turns and afterward place it on the new heating stone. Rapidly shower the batter done with water and afterward cowl with a hot cooking top. Prepare for twenty minutes. Following 20 minutes, start the simmering top and turn down the broiler to 400F/204C degrees. Keep heating for concerning ten extra minutes, turning most of the way for sautéing. Take out your bread and spot it on a cooling rack. At that point flip the stove duplicate to 425F/218C and place the cooking top back in to preheat for 5 - 10 minutes till the following portion is set up to go in.

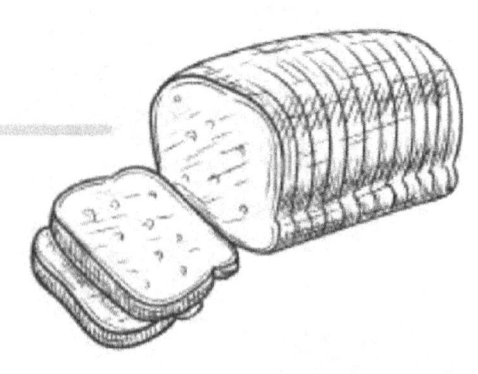

- Cool the bread and eat with ongoing margarine. Sourdough bread is consistently at its best the primary day heated. This portion is horrendously decent sprinkled with sesame or poppy seeds. Make an egg wash of 1 egg overpowered with one Tablespoon of water and spread this over the mixture before cutting. Sprinkle the seeds over the egg-washed mixture and afterward slice. Proceed with the preparation.

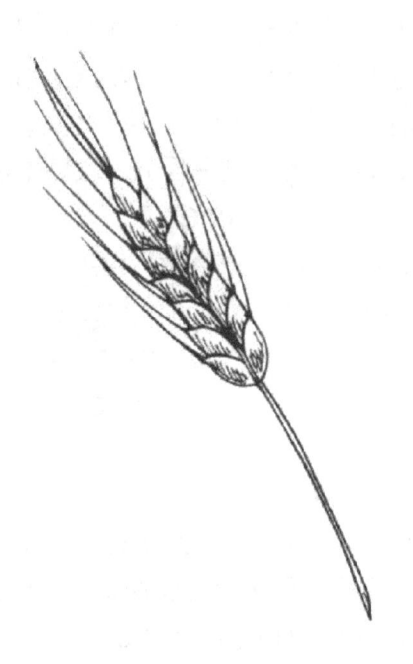

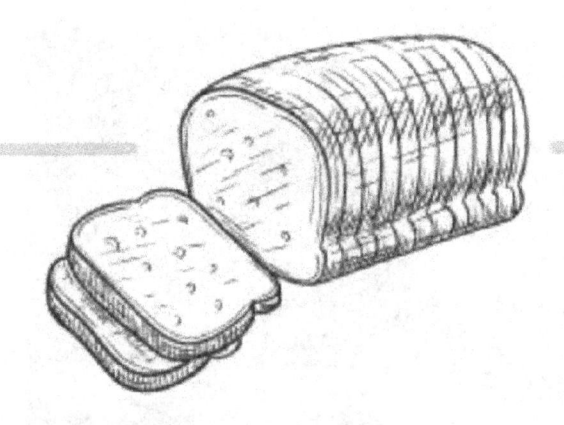

Rosemary Potato Sourdough

Ingredients:

- 2 mugs Bread Flour – 9 Ounce
- 1 mug vigorous sourdough starter – 9 Ounce
- 1 one-fourth mugs water – 10 Ounce
- half mug Rye Flour – 1.8 – Ounce

Instructions:

- Combine all ingredients, except salt, simply until incorporated, and then allow the dough to rest for 20 minutes (dough autolysis). After dough autolysis, stir in salt and then combine dough at low speed for four minutes.

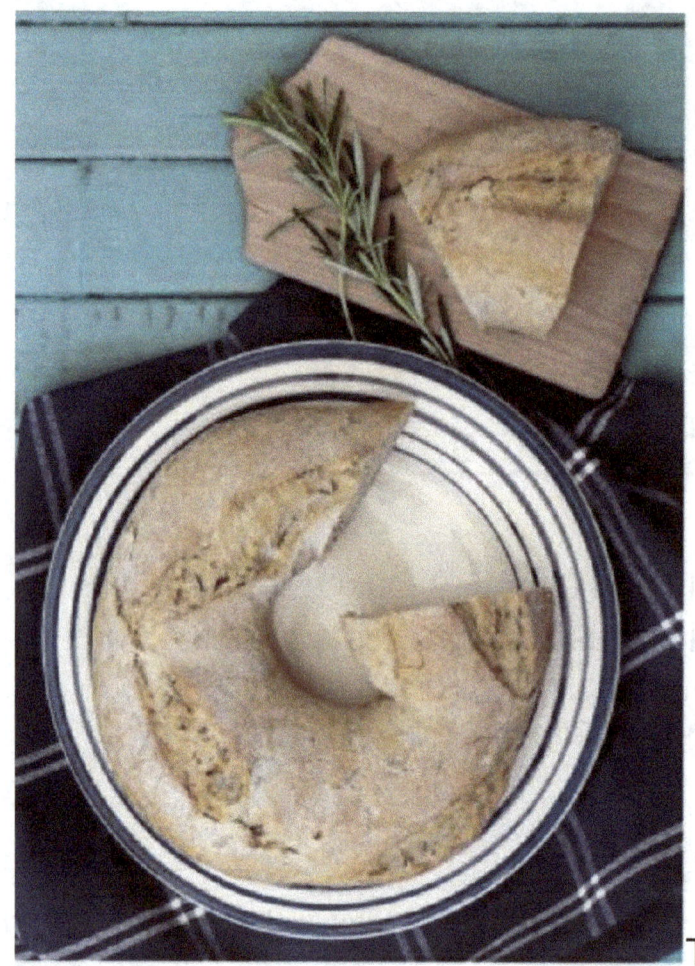

- Then let the dough bulk ferment (1st rise) for 4 – six hours or till doubled. Stir the dough down or fold it once each hour. After bulk fermentation, pour out the dough onto a gently floured surface and knead enough to gather into a ball.
- Divide the dough into two pieces. Form loaf into the general shape you want and then allow the dough to rest for 5 – 10 minutes (bench rest).

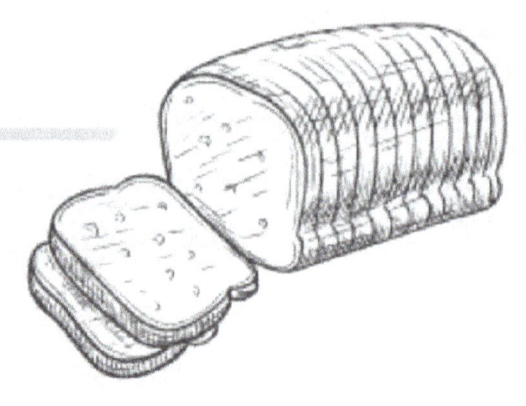

Stagger the shaping of every loaf 30 minutes apart. Place loaves in bannetons and let proof for one-half to 2 hours or when loaves are about one-half times their original size.

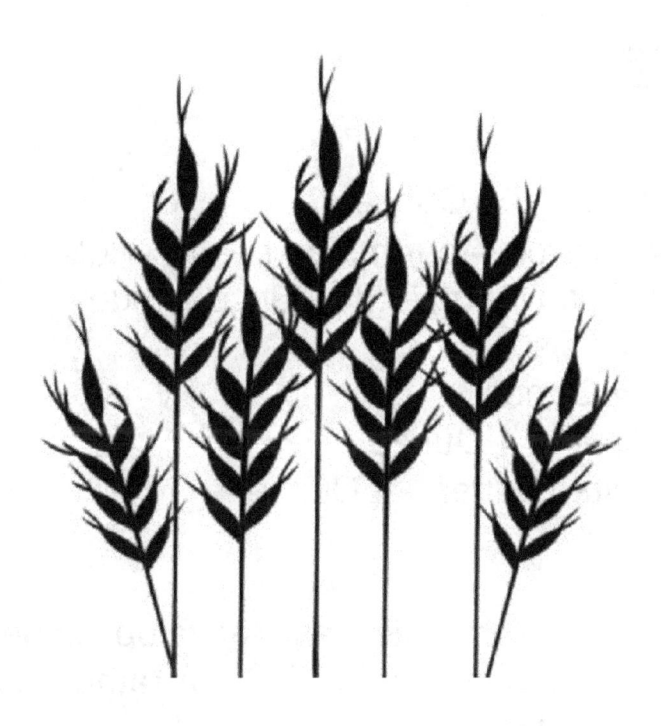

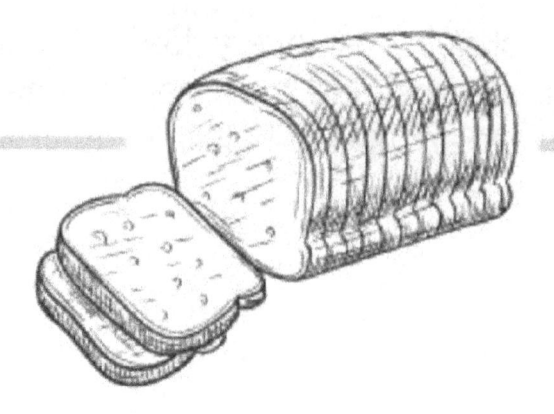

Sourdough Hercules

Ingredients:

- 2 large beaten eggs – 3.5 Ounce
- Honey – 2 Ounce (or one-fourth mug sugar) – 1.8
- Ounce 2 tsp vanilla flavoring – .30 Ounce 1 mug
- sourdough starter
- half mug water - 4 Ounce
- half mug canned milk - 4 Ounce
- half mug oil or melted butter – 4 Ounce

Instructions:

- Draw out your Able skiver dish and develop some Able skivers. They are a particularly lovely treat rather than the typical flapjacks or waffles.
- On the off chance that you at any point locate a decent solid metal Able skiver container… get it! Mine is old and all-around prepared, the base has some surface rust which will not fall off except if I get a metal scrubber in there, that I will not as it will be back in the blink of an eye in my environment. It has seven little dejections to load up with the player.
- The container must be hot like an iron where a drop of water sizzles and hops. Oil the minuscule dishes. At that point fill each downturn with the player and stand by until the Able skiver sets practically nothing.

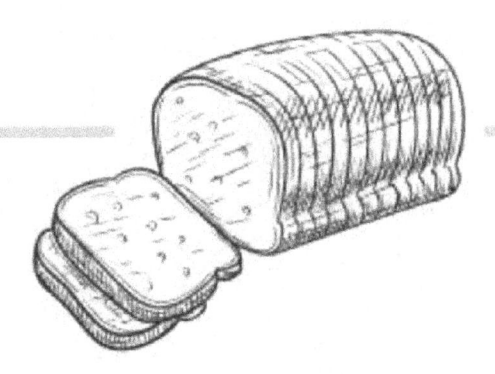

- At that point you are taking a slender sharp-pointed blade or an impeccable sewing needle and push it into the hitter to the underside of the little bowl, you use the blade and pull the Able skiver around, so it is setting mostly up and the player in the center spills out and begins cooking on the lower part of the bowl. As you keep on turning the Able skiver while it's cooking, you produce a ball with an empty center.

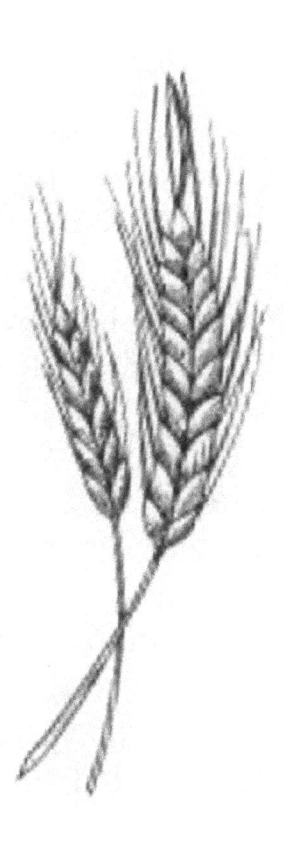

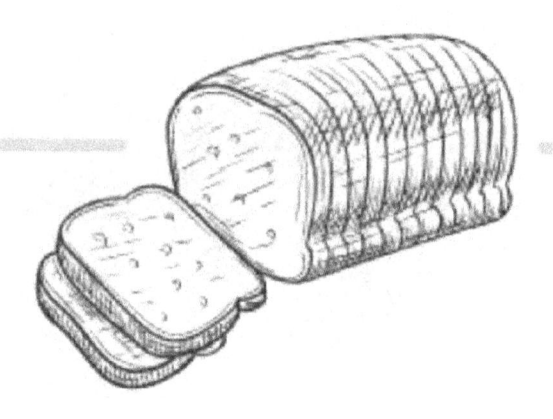

Sunrise Sourdough

Ingredients:

- 1/3 mug Rye flour- 1.2 Ounce
- 1/3 mug Whole Wheat flour-1.4
- Ounce 1 mug active starter
- 2 mugs water -16 Ounce
- 3 mugs bread flour- 13.5 Ounce

Instructions:

- Join the fixings together until all-around consolidated and afterward let the mixture rest for 20 minutes (batter autolysis). After mixture autolysis, add the salt and Combine the butter at low speed for yet one more moment.
- Allow this mixture to confirmation until 6 pm. At that point structure portions and put them into the cooler short-term in plastic-covered crates or bowls. The next morning remove portions independently, amazing 30 minutes separated. At that point let the batter warm-up and verification for around 2 - a couple of of.5 hours or when the mixture increments in size concerning one-half times.
- At that point cut the mixture while still on the strip, slide into the new preheated 450F/232.2C degree broiler onto a hot heating stone, splash the batter once with water rapidly, and afterward cover with a cooking top that has conjointly been preheated in the stove. Prepare for 20 minutes.
- After 20minutes, start the broiling cover and turn down the broiler to 400F/204.4C degrees. Keep heating for 18 - 25

additional minutes or till your bread thermometer peruses 200 205F/93-96C.

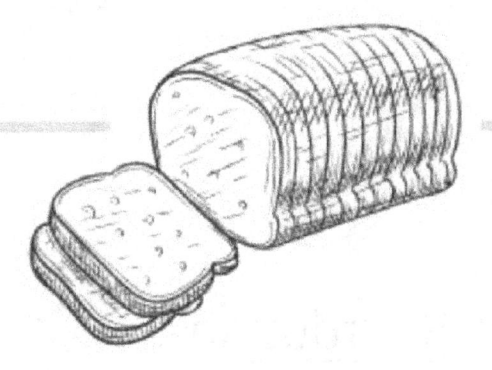

Turn the portion partially through the last heating period for cooking. Cool. For the accompanying portion, turn the stove copy and spot the cooking cover back in to preheat for 5 - ten minutes or until the portion is set up to go in.

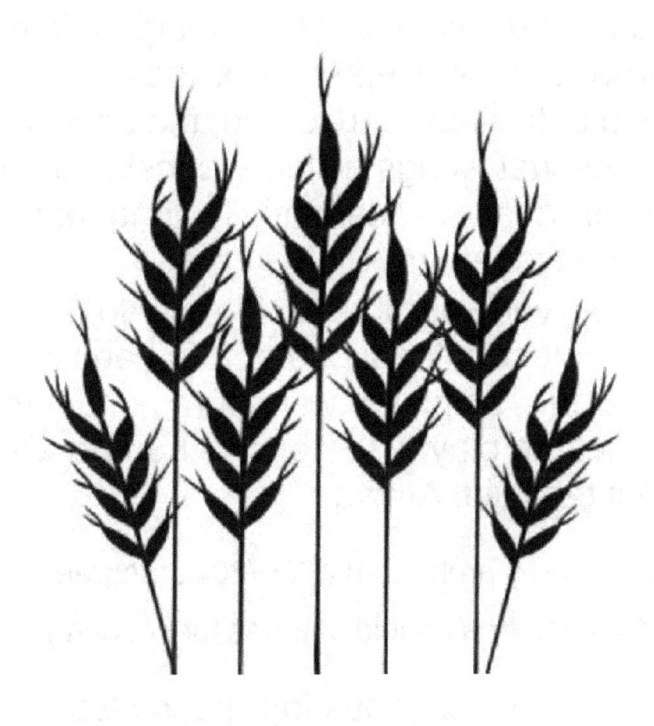

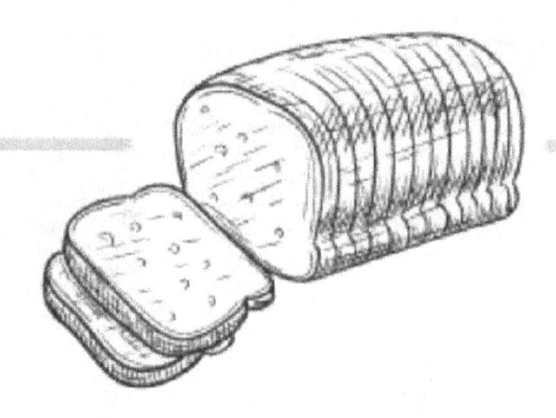

Honey Butter Sourdough

Ingredients:

- half mug of melted butter cooled to lukewarm – 4 Ounce/113g
- 3 large eggs (beaten slightly before putting in Mixer) – 5.2 Ounce/147g
- 1/4 mug of honey or malt syrup – 3Ounce/85g
- 3 mugs of sourdough starter (at 166% hydration) – 27Ounce/765g
- 1 mug evaporated milk (or half & half milk) – 8Ounce/226g

Instructions:

- Consolidate these fixings along barely enough to join them. In a different bowl Combine ether. Mix those dry fixings along with a spoon until all-around joined and afterward add the dry fixings to the wet fixings which are inside the Mixer. Turn on the Mixer and mix essentially long enough to consolidate all fixings together.
- At that point empty your cornbread hitter into a gigantic seventeen mug Bundt or cake dish that has been splashed with skillet oil or lubed. The player will return up to three/4 of the skillet sides. I let the player set for one hour to allow the cornmeal to ingest the fluid. At that

point I heated the bread during a preheated 400F/204C degree broiler for fifty minutes, turning the container a couple of times for sautéing.

- This formula can make a monstrous four-pound four Ounce

portion of cornbread, cut the sums down the middle for a more modest Bundt dish.

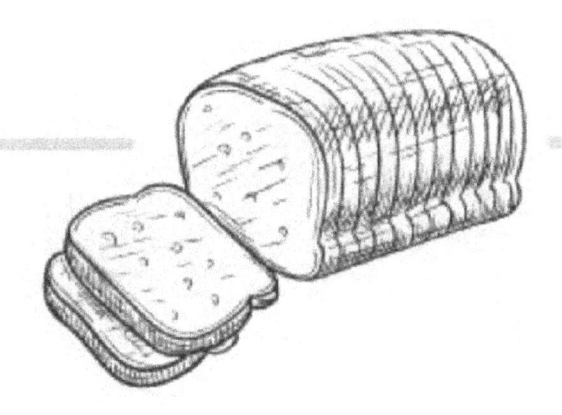

Lentil with Wheat Flour Sourdough
Ingredients:

- With a hand blender, Combine the lentils until they begin to resemble flour. Add water and spelled flour. Pour the
- mixture into a jar with a tight-fitting lid.
- half mug (100 ml) dried green lentils
- half mug (100 ml) water, room
- temperature 1 tbsp spelled flour, sifted
- half mug (100 ml) water, room temperature

Instructions:

- Add the water. Combine well and let stand among the glass jar for two-four days. Stir in the mornings and evenings. The starter is prepared when the Mixture starts to bubble. From this point on, all you've got need to strive to value is "feed" the dough thus that it retains its flavor and talent to ferment.
- If you allow the sourdough in the refrigerator, you must feed it once each week with 0.5 mugs (a hundred ml) water and one mug (a hundred g) lentil flour, that's corresponding to approximately? mug (a hundred and fifty ml) lentils. If you keep the sourdough at room temperature, it should be fed each day, ideally. The consistency should resemble thick porridge. If

you've got sourdough leftover, you'll freeze it in containers that hold a mug.

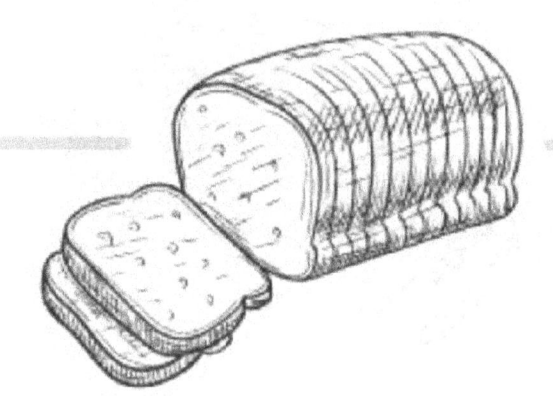

Wheaten Houston Sourdough

Ingredients:

- Water 2 1/2 mugs (11 1/4 ounces)
- 2 mug sourdough flour, divided
- 1 teaspoon kosher salt
- 1 tablespoon olive oil
- 4 ounces (by weight)
- sourdough starter
- 1 mug (4 1/2 ounces) rye flour
- 1 1/4 mugs room temperature
- Nonstock baking spray

Instructions:

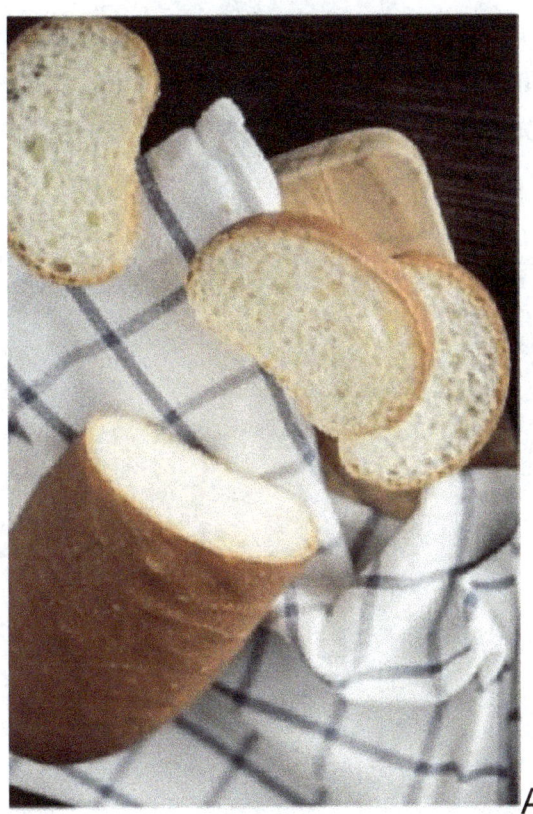

- Add the leftover 3/four mug water, the sourdough flour, salt, and olive oil to the bowl containing the sourdough starter Mixture. Ply with the batter snare of the Stand Mixer or consolidate by hand until the mixture gets smooth. The batter will be wet and tacky, yet don't be enticed to add extra flour. Splash a 9 x 5-inch portion dish with a preparing shower and move the mixture to the skillet.

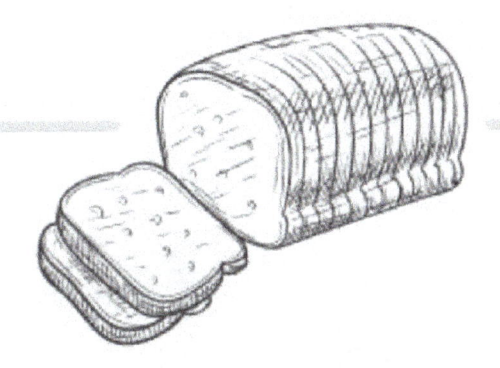

- With delicately lubed fingertips, spread the mixture in the container to even it out. Cover the dish with cling wrap or spot the whole skillet in an incredibly enormous plastic sack and tie the open completion shut. Refrigerate the sourdough short-term or as long as 24 hours before preparing.

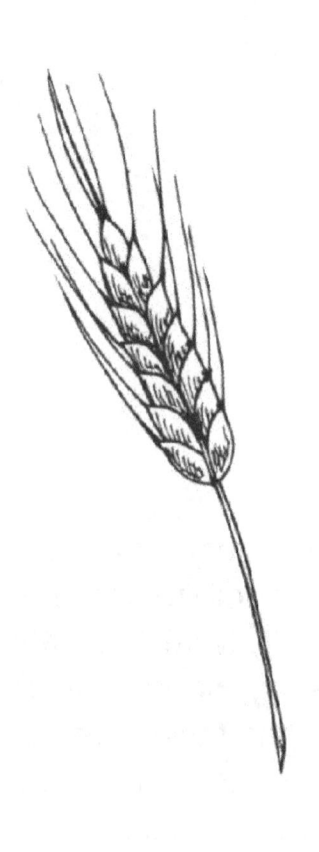

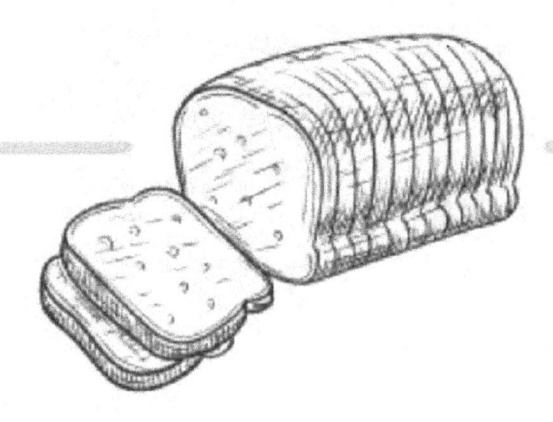

Hoochie Mama Sourdough

Ingredients:

- 1 tablespoon sugar
- 1 teaspoon kosher salt
- 1 teaspoon olive oil
- 1 1/4 mugs room temperature water
- 2 1/4 tsp active dry yeast
- 3 mugs (13 1/2 ounces) sourdough
- flour, plus more as needed
- Rice flour (for dusting the loaves)

Instructions:

- Join the entirety of the fixings aside from the oil and rice flour and ply by hand (consolidate first in a monster bowl, at that point end up and manipulate) or in a very stand Mixer fitted with the batter snare, till the mixture is all around joined and somewhat less shaggy. You don't wish it to get flexible, anyway, it should be very much joined and intelligent. Sprinkle the olive oil into a gallon-size nothing-high plastic pack and move the mixture to the sack. (Flour your hands first, as the mixture is tacky.)
- Squish the batter around inside the pack to cover it with olive oil. Even though the mixture is very tacky, the oil will return among it and the plastic sack as you give it a light back rub. Extract the air from the pack, seal, and refrigerate at least for the time being. This mixture improves with age, so you'll leave it in the fridge a further day, on the off chance that you like.

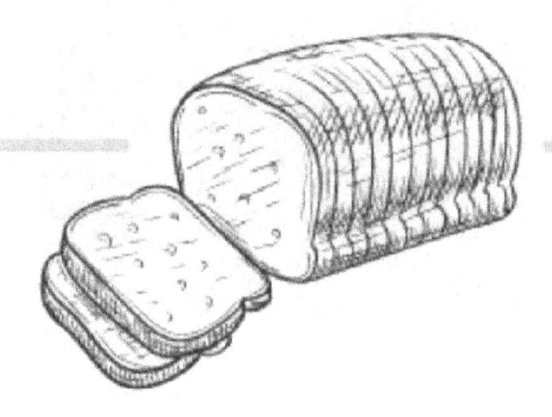

Molasses Wheat Sourdough

Ingredients:

- 2 Tbsp dark Molasses – 1.4 Ounce/39.7g
- 1.2 Ounce/34g (.25 mug) wheat bran, softened with 2 Ounce/56.7g
- boiling water, then cool
- 2 one-fourth mugs Bread flour – 10.1 Ounce/ 286g
- 5 mugs Whole Wheat flour – 21 Ounce/595g
- 1.5 mugs vigorous starter
- 1 mug water – 8 Ounce
- third-fourth mug strong room-temperature coffee – 6 Ounce/170g
- 2 Tbsp Oil – 1 Ounce/28g
- 3 half tsp of salt - .7 Ounce/19.8g (add after dough autolysis)

Instructions:

- Join the fixings on a medium speed basically till consolidated, this takes about a couple of - three minutes. At that point grant the batter to autolyze (rest) for twenty minutes. After autolysis, add at that point consolidate mixture on low speed for concerning 2 minutes. Allow the batter to mass mature (that simply implies that the essential ascent) for four - vi hours until multiplied. After mass maturation, spill out the batter onto a delicately floured (wheat flour) surface and massage various occasions, at that point accumulate into a ball. Gap the batter into 2 enormous things.
- Structure portions into the general structure you might want and

afterward license the batter to rest for five minutes (seat rest). After sidelining structure portions into their last shapes and spot them into the sealing crates, or dish which is fixed with sealing materials if you might want (Bannetons don't should be lined).

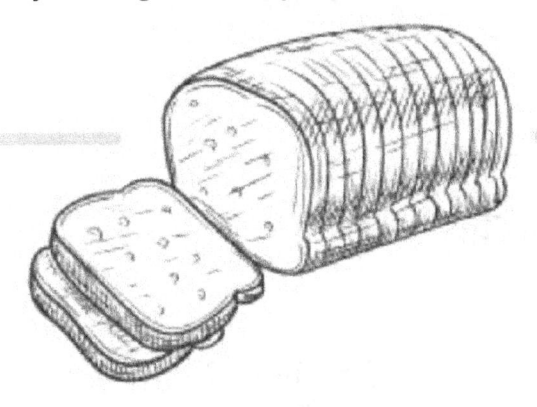

Refrigerate for the time being. Next morning, discard the batter staggered for forty minutes separated and grant the mixture to heat up and confirmation. At the point when the mixture is arranged and feels effervescent and springy however not droopy, that point, taking the main portion to sprinkle the top (actually the base) with semolina or entire grain flour and turn the batter out onto a strip of level heating sheet.

- At that point cut the mixture while it is as yet on the strip, slide the batter into the hot preheated 450F/232.2C degree broiler onto a hot heating stone, shower the mixture once with water rapidly, and afterward cover with a simmering top that has conjointly been preheated in the stove.
- Heat for twenty minutes. After 20minutes, jump out the simmering cover and flip down the stove to 400F/204.4C degrees. Keep heating for 18 - 25 additional minutes or until your bread thermometer peruses 200 205F/93 96C. Turn the portion part of the way through the last preparing sum for cooking. Cool. For the accompanying portion, flip the broiler keep a duplicate and spot the simmering top back in to preheat for 5 - ten minutes or until the portion is set up to go in. Cool and get delighted from slathered with the ongoing spread. This bread makes awesome toast.

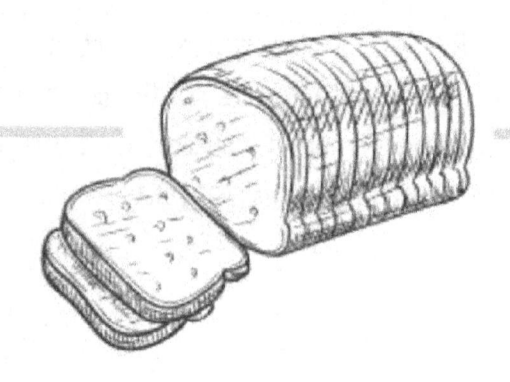

Francisco Sourdough

Ingredients:

- 1/2 mug (3 ounces) semolina flour
- 1 teaspoon kosher salt
- 1 tablespoon olive oil
- 1 1/4 mugs room temperature water
- 2 1/4 tsp active dry yeast
- 1 tablespoon sugar
- 2 1/2 mugs (11 1/4 ounces) sourdough
- 3/4 mug sunflower seeds,
- Nonstock baking spray
- Egg wash (1 egg beaten with

Instructions:

- Join the entirety of the fixings aside from the egg wash and a held one/four cup of sunflower seeds and ply by hand (Combine first in an enormous bowl, at that point flip out and massage) or in an incredibly stand Mixer fitted with the batter snare until the mixture is flexible. Cover the bowl with saran wrap and let the mixture ascend till it has multiplied in size, around 1 hour in a warm space. In the interim, splash four smaller than expected portion skillet (53/four x 3 inches) with a heating shower.
- Flip the batter out onto a delicately floured surface and gap it into four equivalents parcels. Working independently, pat it into a harsh five-inch sq., at that point roll the batter, jellyroll style, to make a fat log. Squeeze the crease and finish shut and place the log, crease viewpoint down, into one among the prepared dishes.

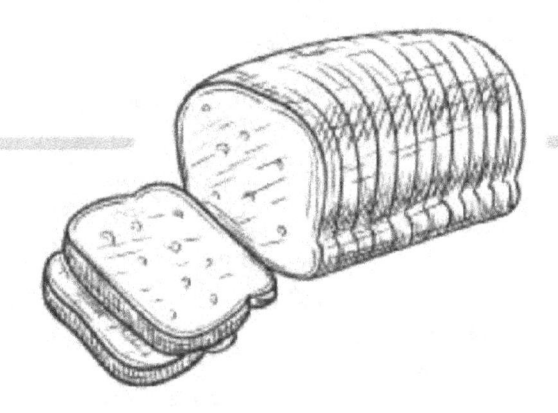

- Proceed with the other three bits of the mixture. Cover the dish with cling wrap or spot them on a heating sheet (for simpler taking care of) and put the whole container in a goliath plastic pack and tie the open end shut. Refrigerate for the time being or up to 24 hours before heating.

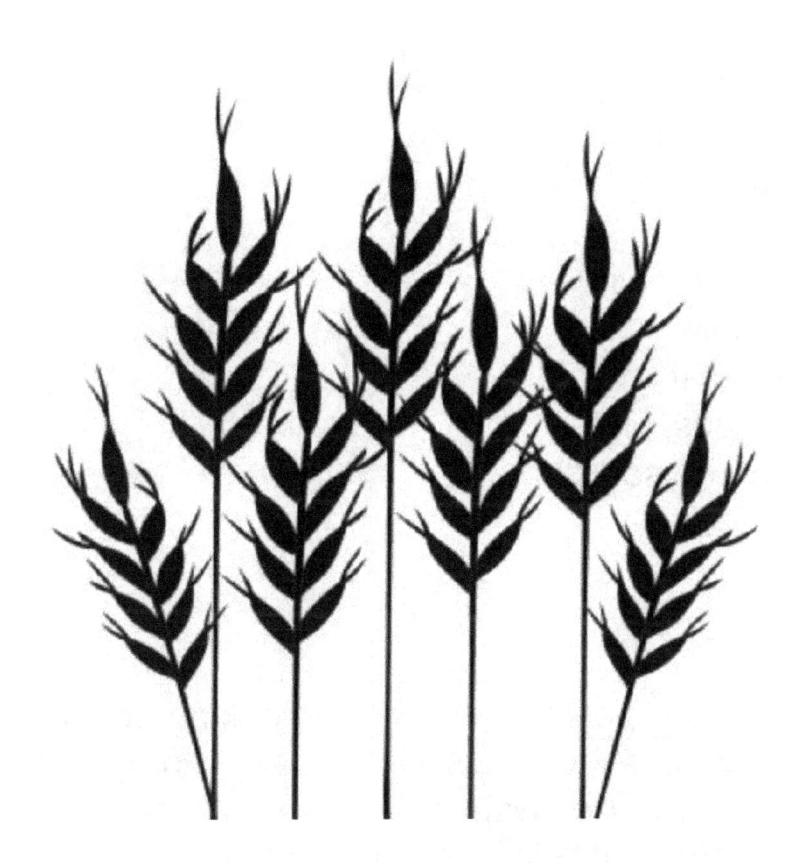

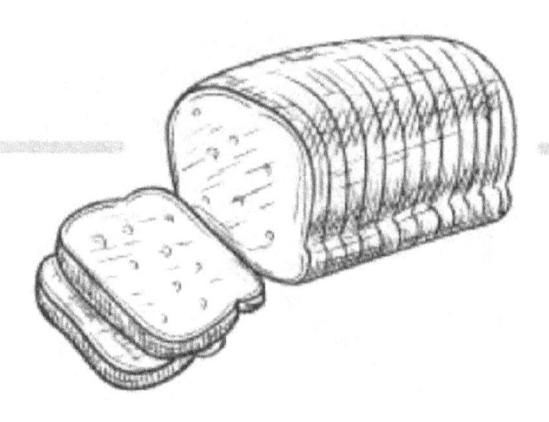

Gluten-Free Nuts sourdough

Ingredients:

- 1 teaspoon kosher salt
- 1/4 mug corn-starch
- 1 tablespoon xanthan gum
- 1/4 mug chopped walnuts
- 1/4 mug sunflower seeds
- 1/4 mug flax seeds
- Nonstock cooking spray
- 2 1/2 mugs (13 3/4 ounces) King
- Arthur Flour gluten-free
- multipurpose flour
- 3 eggs
- 1 1/2 mugs room temperature
- 1/2 mug nonfat dry milk
- 2 1/4 tsp active dry yeast
- 1/4 mug sesame seeds, plus
- more for the top of the sourdough
- 2 tbsp unsalted butter,
- at room temperature

Instructions:

- Shower a nine x 5-inch portion dish with a cooking splash (don't utilize preparing shower, which contains flour). Or then again brush the skillet with cooking oil, if you like. Consolidate every one of the fixings in a Stand Mixer fitted with the oar connection.

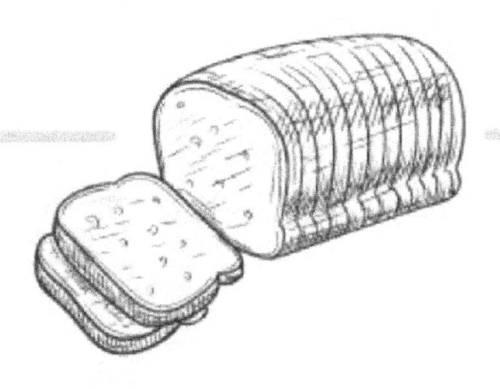

- You will likewise join this in a huge bowl with a hand Mixer. Beat for five minutes. The surface will not resemble sourdough batter; however, you'll see the mixture start to appear to be next to no gluey—like pureed potatoes that have turned out badly.

- Move the batter to the readied skillet and smooth out the top with saturated fingers. Cover the skillet with saran wrap or spot the dish in an enormous plastic pack and tie the open end shut. Refrigerate the batter for the time being or up to 24 hours.

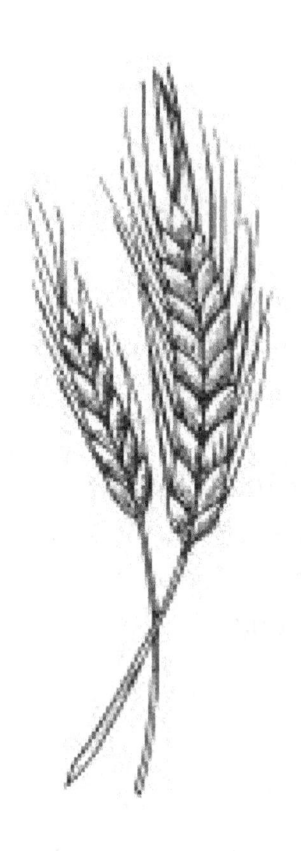

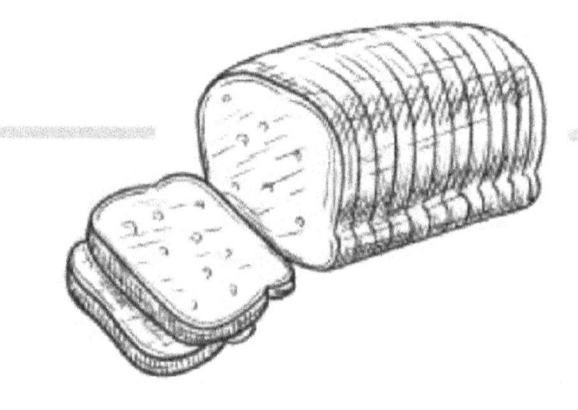

Yeast wood Sourdough

Ingredients:

- 1.5 mug Bread Flour – 6.75 Ounce
- half mug Spelt or Whole Wheat Flour – 2.1
- Ounce 1 mug vigorous sourdough starter 1
- mug water – 8.0 Ounce
- 1/4 mug Rye Flour – 1.0 – Ounce

Instructions:

- Consolidate all fixings along just as salt for 3 minutes. At that point let the mixture age for in regards to four hours more. After mass maturation, spill out the mixture onto a tenderly floured surface and ply enough to gather into a ball. Gap the mixture into two things. Shape portion into the general shape you need and afterward grant the mixture to rest for 5 – ten minutes (seat rest).
- After sidelining shape portions into their last shapes and put them into sealed containers or lined bannetons. Spot bushels into a plastic pack and the fridge short-term. Toward the beginning of the day, seize the portions piecemeal concerning thirty minutes separated, and permit the batter to conclusive verification for around two hours. At that point cut, splash once, and cover with a cooking top that has been preheated in a 450F/232C degree broiler. Prepare for 20 minutes.
- At that point, come out the cooking top, being cautious about the new steam. At that point flip down the stove to 425F/218C degrees and keep preparing for concerning 15-twenty extra minutes or until your bread thermometer peruses 200-205F/93 96C, turning most of the way for cooking. Cool. Eat with loads of margarine.

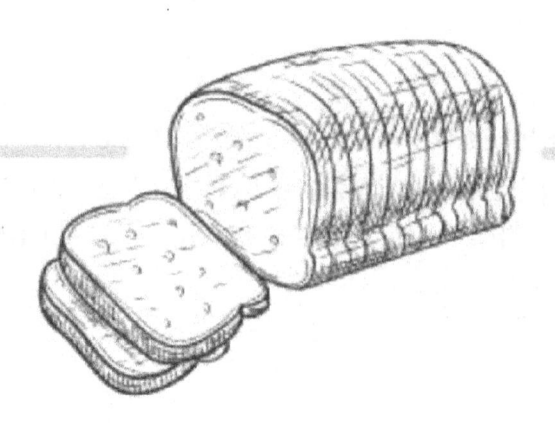

Sourdine Sourdough

Ingredients:

- 3 Mugs All-Purpose flour (or substitute half mug Whole Wheat flour for a half mug of AP flour, if using Honey instead of Malt syrup, then you can have Honey Whole Wheat Flapjacks). – 13.2 Ounce/374g
- 1 Tablespoon Baking Powder - .5 Ounce/14g
- half mug melted, cooled butter – 4 Ounce/113g 1 mug evaporated milk – 8 Ounce/226g half mug water – 4 Ounce/113g
- 2 mugs vigorous sourdough starter
- 1 generous Tablespoon of Malt syrup (or Honey) – 1 Ounce/28g
- 1 teaspoon Baking Soda - .16 Ounce/4.5g
- 1 teaspoon salt – .2 Ounce/5.7g

Instructions:

- Presently add the dry fixings to the wet fixings and mix along tenderly. Allow the player to set for concerning ten – 15 minutes to permit the flour to retain the fluids, and secure your iron keen and hot, concerning 375F/190C degrees. Daintily oil the frying pan. Iron your hotcakes till one aspect is effervescent and the edges are marginally dry, at that point flip once and frying pan on the other feature.
- Present with stores of new margarine and Maple syrup (we will in general add Malt syrup to our Maple syrup for extra flavor). Persuade arranged to be requested a great deal of! This formula makes a clump of in regards to twenty hotcakes for a goliath

family or a lot of second helpings. So cut the sums down the middle for a more modest group.

CPSIA information can be obtained
at www.ICGtesting.com
Printed in the USA
BVHW061054230621
610291BV00003B/324